Practical Guide to Diabetes Management

SECOND EDITION

Practical Guide to Diabetes Management

SECOND EDITION

William T. Cefalu, M.D.
Associate Professor
Department of Medicine
Endocrine, Diabetes & Metabolism Unit
University of Vermont College of Medicine
Burlington, Vermont

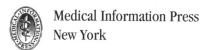
Medical Information Press
New York

Contents

INTRODUCTION

The second edition of *Practical Guide to Diabetes Management* has been significantly revised to provide practical, up-to-date information on diabetes in an easy-to-use format. Serving as a quick-reference guide to diabetes diagnosis and treatment, this book allows physicians to keep pace with the latest developments. Staying abreast of this information is vital to patient care: An estimated 16 million people in the United States have diabetes,[1] of whom 5.4 million have undiagnosed diabetes. Most notably, diabetes is the seventh leading cause of death, with more than 190,000 deaths resulting from the disease and its complications in 1996.[1]

Although diabetes takes a terrible toll on patients and their families, the long-term outlook has improved dramatically. Physicians, along with a team of nurses, diabetes educators, dietitians, exercise physiologists, and other health care providers, can help change the course of this disease and reduce its burden. Toward that end, each chapter in this book offers practical advice for managing the care of both patients with type 1 diabetes and those with type 2 diabetes. Cross-referenced throughout, the text allows the physician to navigate easily through a subject to provide answers to patients' questions. Charts and bulleted lists present needed information in an easily retrievable format.

Starting with a discussion of the pathophysiology and natural history of the disease in Chapter 1, the book moves on to cover up-to-date American Diabetes Association (ADA) guidelines for the diagnosis of diabetes, including the revised criteria for diagnosing gestational diabetes, in Chapter 2. A completely revised Chapter 3 reviews the complications of diabetes in light of data from the Diabetes Control and Complications Trial (DCCT) and the United Kingdom Prospective Diabetes Study (UKPDS), with particular emphasis on the implications of these trials for minimizing diabetes complications. In Chapter 4, practical advice on designing a plan for diabetes management is given; diet and exercise are discussed in Chapter 5. Chapters 6 and 7 have been updated to include the latest oral therapeutic agents and insulin formulations, respectively. A heavily revised Chapter 8 now covers standards of care as outlined by the ADA, including new information on lipid management. The last chapter, Chapter 9, describes the most recent innovations in diabetes research, with information on needleless glucose monitors, β-cell transplants, and noninvasive forms of insulin delivery, among other advances. Finally, the Appendix contains an extensive list of patient resources.

■ What Is Diabetes Mellitus?

In 1889, two German scientists accidentally discovered that a dog whose pancreas they had removed for study passed sugar in its urine. Eventually, Joseph von Mering and Oskar Minkowski proved that a pancreatic secretion controls the body's use of sugar, and in 1921, the secretion was isolated. It turned out to be the hormone insulin, so named because it is produced by clusters of isolated, or insular, pancreatic cells, the islets of Langerhans. Within a year, scientists were testing purified extracts of beef pancreas on humans with diabetes, and, in 1923, John J. R. MacLeod and his colleague Frederick Banting of the University of Toronto won the Nobel Prize in medicine for their work. Thirty years later, Frederick Sanger of Cambridge University defined the amino acid sequence of bovine insulin and collected a Nobel Prize in chemistry.[2]

■ Who Is Affected by Diabetes Mellitus?

As mentioned above, according to the United States National Institute of Diabetes and Digestive and Kidney Diseases (NIDDK), as many as 16 million people in the United States have diabetes: 8.1 million women, 7.5 million men, and about 100,000 youths and children under the age of 20 years. Nearly one third of these individuals remain unaware of their condition, and each year 798,000 new cases are diagnosed. Because of an aging and increasingly obese population, diabetes has risen an alarming 700% in the United States since the 1970s. Even adolescents are now found to have type 2 diabetes, which originally was more often associated with middle-aged adults.[1,3]

Certain ethnic groups—African Americans, Hispanics, and Native Americans—suffer a disproportionately higher incidence of the disease and its related morbidity. Diabetes costs $98 billion a year in direct and indirect medical costs tallied in disability, work loss, and premature mortality.[1]

■ Incidence of Other Diseases Associated with Diabetes

Often, the first hint that a patient has diabetes is when he or she develops complications, which are sometimes life-threatening. The following statistics are from the NIDDK and the ADA:[1,3]

- Cardiovascular disease, the leading cause of diabetes-related deaths, is two to four times more common in people with diabetes.
- Approximately 60–65% of people with diabetes have hypertension.
- The risk of stroke is two to four times higher in people with diabetes.
- Diabetes is the leading cause of new cases of blindness among adults between 20 and 74 years of age.
- Diabetes accounts for 40% of new cases of end-stage renal disease.

- About 60–70% of people with diabetes have mild to severe forms of nerve damage, a major contributing cause of amputation.

- More than half of lower-limb amputations in the United States occur among people with diabetes.

- Between 1993 and 1995, the average number of amputations performed each year among people with diabetes was 67,000.

- Between 3% and 5% of pregnancies among women with diabetes result in the death of the newborn.

- In the absence of preconception care, the prevalence of major congenital birth defects in infants of mothers with diabetes is about 10%.

- The prevalence of impotence in men over the age of 50 with diabetes has been reported to be as high as 50–60%.

■ References

1. American Diabetes Association. Diabetes Info: Diabetes Facts and Figures. Available at: http://www.diabetes.org/ada/c20f.html. Accessed September 8, 2000.
2. Kelley DB, ed-in-chief. *American Diabetes Association Complete Guide to Diabetes*. Alexandria, Va: American Diabetes Association; 1996:27–29.
3. National Institute of Diabetes and Digestive and Kidney Diseases (NIDDK). Diabetes Statistics. National Diabetes Information Clearinghouse. Available at: http://www.niddk.nih.gov/health/diabetes/pubs/dmstats/dmstats.html. Accessed September 8, 2000.

Pathophysiology

■ Physiology of Glucose Metabolism

The pancreas plays an integral role in glucose metabolism. In this organ are scattered more than 1 million clusters of islets of Langerhans, and β-cells within the islets produce and store insulin, whereas α-cells manufacture and store the counteracting hormone, glucagon. As ingested carbohydrates are converted into glucose and enter the bloodstream, β-cells react to the rising serum glucose levels and increase insulin output. Insulin, the body's chief regulator of glucose metabolism, attaches to receptor sites on the surface of cells. When insulin binds to these receptors, the insulin receptor initiates a chain of cellular signals that ultimately results in a regulated movement of glucose transport proteins from inside the cell to the cellular membrane. This facilitates glucose entry into the cell. With the exception of cells in the brain, lens of the eye, renal medulla, and red blood cells, glucose cannot enter a cell unless insulin binds to its receptor.

Glucose not burned for energy is converted by the liver and muscles to glycogen and stored for future use. When blood glucose levels return to normal after a meal (postprandial), insulin secretion decreases. If an individual has not eaten for several hours, a drop in blood glucose stimulates the α-cells into secreting glucagon, which in turn signals the liver to convert stored glycogen back into glucose and secrete it into the bloodstream.

Normally, the islets of Langerhans perform a perfect balancing act, monitoring blood glucose levels and releasing insulin or glucagon in the appropriate amounts. They maintain a steady-state glucose level by acting in concert with the liver and peripheral tissues. But in diabetes, the disease process breaks the loop at one of several points. Most notably in type 1 diabetes, antibodies mount an immunologic attack on β-cells during a preclinical period of several years. Before hyperglycemia ever occurs, at least 80–90% of the β-cells' function must fail.[1]

■ Natural History of Diabetes Mellitus

Diabetes mellitus results either from an absolute deficiency of insulin caused by a pancreas that no longer produces insulin or from a relative deficiency of insulin in the presence of an increased demand (i.e., insulin resistance). The disease manifests in three main forms. (See Chapter 2 for more details on the new nomenclature.)

TYPE 1 DIABETES

Type 1 diabetes, formerly referred to as insulin-dependent diabetes mellitus (IDDM), constitutes 10% of all diabetes cases. In most instances, this disease is diagnosed in children and adolescents; each year, doctors diagnose 12,000 new cases of type 1 diabetes in patients younger than 19 years of age, making it the most common chronic disorder in American children.[2]

Type 1 diabetes, an autoimmune disease, most often results from antibody attacks on pancreatic β-cells, resulting in irreparable damage. Some evidence indicates that environmental factors, possibly including viruses such as coxsackie B or mumps, may play a role in this process. Type 1 diabetes often seems to emerge clinically in winter and spring months, presumably after exposure to these viruses. Regardless of the underlying cause, however, loss of β-cell function can be detected from months to years before the onset of type 1 diabetes,[3] an observation that has prompted the initiation of the Diabetes Prevention Trial–Type 1 (DPT-1). This study is aimed at determining whether insulin can delay or prevent diabetes by altering the immune process destroying β-cells.[4] (See Chapter 9.)

Although nearly all people with type 1 diabetes carry genetic markers on chromosomes 6 and 11, 70–80% of cases occur sporadically. Among identical twins in whom one twin contracts type 1 diabetes, only about half of the second twins will be affected. This observation suggests that a genetic predisposition combined with exposure to an environmental factor might be necessary to cause the disease.[3]

TYPE 2 DIABETES

Type 2 diabetes, formerly referred to as non-insulin-dependent diabetes mellitus (NIDDM), accounts for nearly 90% of diagnosed diabetes cases and for almost all of those that go undiagnosed. This disease, sometimes referred to as adult-onset diabetes, usually occurs in adults older than 40 years, with most cases occurring in adults older than 55 years.[1] Obese patients, particularly those with abdominal fat or "central obesity," are at increased risk for type 2 diabetes.

The natural history of type 2 diabetes is complex (Figure 1-1). Most of these patients do produce insulin, but because of a combination of factors, including insulin resistance and β-cell dysfunction, there is a relative insulin deficiency and a compromised ability to metabolize glucose. Insulin resistance is a condition in which an increased amount of insulin is required to transport glucose across cell membranes. The causes of β-cell dysfunction in type 2 diabetes are still under investigation. Generally, however, the pancreatic

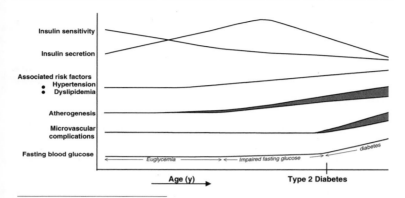

Figure 1-1. Proposed metabolic observations in the natural history of type 2 diabetes. (Reprinted from Cefalu WT. Insulin resistance. In: Leahy JL, Clark NG, Cefalu WT, eds. *Medical Management of Diabetes Mellitus.* New York, NY: Marcel Dekker, Inc; 2000:57–75, with permission.)

islets in patients with type 2 diabetes are smaller than those of normal individuals.[5] Furthermore, under steady-state conditions, islets from type 2 patients produce less insulin than do those from healthy people.[5] Weight loss and exercise may increase the effectiveness of insulin in the peripheral tissues and serve as cornerstones for treatment regimens. (See Chapter 5.)

The progression from normal glucose tolerance to frank diabetes seems to occur in individuals with a genetic susceptibility who exhibit a gradual decline in β-cell function along with insulin resistance. In this early prediabetic stage, normal or near-normal glycemia is achieved because of compensatory hyperinsulinemia. However, when β-cell function can no longer compensate for insulin resistance, hyperglycemia is observed clinically.[6] Results of the landmark United Kingdom Prospective Diabetes Study (UKPDS) established that there is a progressive decline in β-cell function in patients with type 2 diabetes no matter what pharmacologic intervention was prescribed initially. Specifically, pancreatic function was estimated to be approximately 50% of normal at diagnosis and continued to decline over the course of study in all treatment groups. This study clearly illustrates the natural history of type 2 diabetes and strongly suggests combination treatment strategies (see Chapter 4) to maintain glycemic control.[7,8]

GESTATIONAL DIABETES

Gestational diabetes is the term given to diabetes that develops during pregnancy, most often between 24 and 28 weeks of gestation, and usually disappears when the pregnancy ends. Approximately 2–5% of pregnant women who had no diabetes prior to pregnancy will develop gestational diabetes.

The causes of gestational diabetes are not fully understood. During pregnancy, circulating hormones can block insulin action. Some investigators believe that unrecognized diabetes may have already been present in such cases, and the weight gain and hormonal fluctuations of pregnancy simply unmasked the disease. Researchers also suspect that the same genes responsible for type 2 diabetes may predispose a woman to gestational diabetes. Women who have had gestational diabetes have a greater risk of developing type 2 diabetes later in life.[9]

■ Final Note

Diabetes mellitus is a complex disorder involving genes, environment, and metabolic defects such as decreased insulin, insulin resistance, and increased gluconeogenesis and lipolysis. The interplay of these factors creates a challenge to clinicians in the management of diabetes.

■ References

1. Kelley DB, ed-in-chief. *American Diabetes Association Complete Guide to Diabetes.* Alexandria, Va: American Diabetes Association; 1996:14.
2. National Institute of Diabetes and Digestive and Kidney Diseases (NIDDK). Insulin-Dependent Diabetes. NIH Publication No. 94-2098, October 1997. Updated February 10, 1997. Available at: http://www.niddk.nih.gov/Insulin DependentDiabetes/InsulinDependentDiabetes.html.
3. Palmer JP, Lernmark Å. Pathophysiology of type 1 (insulin-dependent) diabetes. In: Porte D Jr, Sherwin RS, eds. *Ellenberg & Rifkin's Diabetes Mellitus.* 5th ed. New York, NY: McGraw-Hill; 1997:455–486.
4. National Institute of Diabetes and Digestive and Kidney Diseases (NIDDK). Conquering diabetes: a strategic plan for the 21st century. 1999. Available at: http://www.EP.NIDDK.NIH.gov/dwg/fr.pdf. Accessed August 21, 2000.
5. Kahn SE, Porte D Jr. The pathophysiology of type 2 (insulin-independent) diabetes mellitus: implications for treatment. In: Porte D Jr, Sherwin RS, eds. *Ellenberg & Rifkin's Diabetes Mellitus.* 5th ed. New York, NY: McGraw-Hill; 1997:487–512.
6. Weyer C, Bogardus C, Mott DM, Pratley RE. The natural history of insulin secretory dysfunction and insulin resistance in the pathogeneses of type 2 diabetes mellitus. *J Clin Invest.* 1999;104:787–794.
7. Turner RC, Cull CA, Frighi V, Holman RR. Glycemic control with diet, sulfonylurea, metformin, or insulin in patients with type 2 diabetes mellitus: progressive requirement for multiple therapies (UKPDS 49). UK Prospective Diabetes Study Group. *JAMA.* 1999;281:2005–2012.
8. Turner RC. The U.K. Prospective Diabetes Study. A review. *Diabetes Care.* 1998;21:C35–C38.
9. National Institute of Diabetes and Digestive and Kidney Diseases (NIDDK). Diabetes Statistics. NIH Publication No. 96-3926. October 1995. Updated August 13, 1997. Available at: http://www.niddk.nih.gov/DiabetesStatistics/DiabetesStatistics.html.

CHAPTER TWO

Diagnosing Diabetes:
The New Guidelines*

An international Expert Committee that was sponsored by the American Diabetes Association (ADA) recently made sweeping recommendations on classification, diagnosis, and wide-scale screening and testing for diabetes mellitus. The committee's work is an update of a similar process last undertaken in 1979 by the National Diabetes Group. Based on a 2-year review of more than 15 years of research, the new recommendations have been widely accepted and will help physicians detect diabetes earlier, possibly resulting in the delay or even the prevention of the onset of complications. The revised cutpoint is based on the observation that cardiovascular, retinal, and renal complications begin earlier than previously thought. Using these criteria, physicians could identify up to two million of the eight million Americans whose adult-onset (type 2) diabetes is undiagnosed.[1]

The Expert Committee recommended eliminating the categories of insulin-dependent diabetes mellitus (IDDM) and non-insulin-dependent diabetes mellitus (NIDDM) because they are based on pharmacologic treatment that can vary considerably and

---

*Sections of this chapter are adapted from American Diabetes Association,[2,3] with permission.

does not indicate the underlying problem. The use of Arabic (type 1 and type 2) rather than Roman (type I and type II) numerals is recommended to prevent confusion. Type II, for example, could be read as "type eleven."[2]

Etiologic Classification of Diabetes Mellitus[3]

1. Type 1 (formerly IDDM)
2. Type 2 (formerly NIDDM)
3. Gestational diabetes mellitus
4. Other specific types

> Genetic defects of β-cell function
>
> Genetic defects in insulin action
>
> Disease of exocrine pancreas
>
> Endocrinopathies
>
> Drug- or chemical-induced
>
> Infections
>
> Uncommon form of immune-mediated disease
>
> Other genetic syndromes associated with diabetes

An individual's diabetes classification may depend on the circumstances at the time of diagnosis. Individuals may not easily fit into a single class.[3]

■ Simplified Testing and Diagnosis[3]

Diabetes can be diagnosed by performing any of these three tests. Results must be confirmed on a subsequent day by any of the three tests.

1. A fasting plasma glucose (FPG) of $\geq$ 126 mg/dl (Table 2-1). Fasting is defined as no caloric intake for at least 8 hours.
2. A casual plasma glucose $\geq$ 200 mg/dl with the classic diabetes symptoms of polyuria, polydipsia, and unexplained weight loss. *Casual* is defined as any time of the day without regard to time since last meal.[3]
3. An oral glucose tolerance test (OGTT) value of $\geq$ 200 mg/dl in the 2-hour plasma glucose sample (2-h PG). The test should be performed using a glucose load equivalent to 75-g anhydrous glucose dissolved in water.[3]

FPG is the preferred test, and the committee recommended moving toward the universal use of FPG for testing and diagnosis because it is easier to administer, faster, more reproducible,[3] more convenient and acceptable to patients, and has a lower cost compared to OGTT.[2]

Warning: The hemoglobin A_{1c} test (also known as HbA_{1c} or glycated hemoglobin) is not recommended for diagnosis. The finger-prick test is also not considered a diagnostic procedure.[1]

	TABLE 2-1 Diagnosing Diabetes	
Stage	Fasting Plasma Glucose (FPG)	Oral Glucose Tolerance Test (OGTT)
Diabetes	FPG $\geq$ 126 mg/dl (7.0 mmol/L)	2-h PG $\geq$ 200 mg/dl
Impaired glucose homeostasis	Impaired fasting glucose (IFG) FPG $\geq$ 110 and < 126 mg/dl	Impaired glucose tolerance (IGT) 2-hour sample (2-h PG) $\geq$ 140 and < 200 mg/dl
Normal	FPG < 110 mg/dl	2-h PG < 140 mg/dl

(Adapted from American Diabetes Association,[3] with permission.)

■ Impaired Glucose Homeostasis

The committee also classified an intermediate state between "normal" and "diabetes." People who fall within this category are at risk for developing diabetes and related complications.[3]

- Upper limit of normal blood glucose: 110 mg/dl on the FPG (see Table 2-1)
- Impaired glucose metabolism or homeostasis is considered a risk factor for future diabetes and cardiovascular disease when the following exists:

  Impaired fasting glucose (IFG), a new category, when FPG ≥ 110 but < 126 mg/dl

  Impaired glucose tolerance (IGT), an existing category, when the OGTT value ≥ 140 but < 200 mg/dl in the 2-hour sample (2-h PG)

People with impaired glucose homeostasis have been shown to be at high risk for developing diabetes and such macrovascular complications as heart attacks and strokes and should be closely monitored.[1] See Chapter 9 for more information on the Diabetes Prevention Program, a major multicenter National Institute of Diabetes and Digestive and Kidney Diseases (NIDDK) clinical trial. The study is designed to determine whether early treatment can prevent or delay development of diabetes in people with impaired glucose homeostasis.[4]

■ Individuals at Risk for Diabetes Mellitus

Individuals at high risk of developing type 1 diabetes can often be identified with serologic evidence of autoimmune pathologic processes in the pancreatic islets and by using genetic markers.[3]

However, testing presumably healthy individuals for the presence of any immune markers outside of a clinical trials setting is not recommended. Although it is still unclear how environmental factors play a role in the development of type 1 diabetes, researchers agree that genetics are not exclusively responsible. Major risk factors for type 1 diabetes are summarized below.[5]

- First degree relative of a person with type 1 diabetes
- Presence of genetic markers such as human leukocyte antigen (HLA), certain tumor necrosis factor (TNF)–α and TNF-β alleles, and other genetic elements
- Immune aspects: presence of islet cell antibodies (ICA), cell-mediated immune mechanisms, release of certain cytokines from the immune cells infiltrating the islet
- Possible environmental factors: exposure to specific drugs or chemicals, early exposure to cow's milk protein, viruses (mumps, coxsackie, and rubella most highly suspected)

Certain attributes or risk factors contribute to the development of type 2 diabetes or are statistically associated with the disease. The greater the number of risk factors, the greater the chance of developing diabetes. Major risk factors for type 2 diabetes are summarized below.[6]

High Risk Factors

- Obesity (more than 20% above ideal body weight or a body mass index [BMI] $\geq$ 27 kg/m^2)
- First-degree relative of a person with diabetes
- Member of a high-risk ethnic group—African American, Hispanic, Native American, Asian
- Age $\geq$ 45 years
- Delivery of a baby weighing more than 9 pounds or diagnosis of gestational diabetes mellitus

- Hypertension (≥ 140/90)
- High-density lipoprotein (HDL) cholesterol level of ≤ 35 mg/dl and/or a triglyceride level of ≥ 250 mg/dl
- IFG or IGT on previous testing

General screening for diabetes may be an appropriate part of routine medical care if one or more of these risk factors are present. On the basis of lack of supporting data, screening of all high-risk individuals is not recommended. The decision to screen should be based on clinical judgment and patient preference. After a negative screening test result, screening of high-risk individuals should be considered at 3-year intervals.[6]

■ Special Recommendations for Pregnant Women[2]

In the past, all pregnant women were tested for gestational diabetes, a disease that complicates about 4% of all pregnancies in the United States. That recommendation has been changed: Pregnant women at low risk do not need to be tested, including those who (1) are less than 25 years old, (2) are of normal body weight, (3) have no family history of diabetes, (4) are not members of an ethnic group with a high prevalence of diabetes, (5) have no history of abnormal glucose tolerance, and (6) have no history of poor obstetric outcome.[7] Women of average risk should be tested between 24 and 28 weeks of gestation. Women with high risk factors should undergo glucose testing as soon as feasible and be retested between 24 and 28 weeks of gestation.[7] A one-step or two-step approach can be used in evaluating for gestational diabetes. In the one-step approach, an OGTT is performed without prior plasma or serum glucose screening. This approach may be cost-effective in high-risk populations.

In the two-step approach, an initial screening of plasma or serum glucose concentration is done 1 hour after a 50-g oral glucose load (glucose challenge test or GCT). In those women who exceed the glucose threshold value of 140 mg/dl with use of the 50-g GCT, a 100-g, 3-hour diagnostic test should be done (Table 2-2).[7] When the two-step approach is used clinically, a glucose threshold value of > 140 mg/dl identifies approximately 80% of women with gestational diabetes mellitus. It has been reported that the yield is further increased to over 90% by using a glucose threshold cutoff of > 130 mg/dl.[7] This test should be done after an overnight fast and 3 days of unrestricted diet.[7] The diagnosis of gestational diabetes requires any two of the four plasma glucose values obtained during the OGTT to meet or exceed the values shown in Table 2-2.

■ A Final Note

Widespread adoption of the new criteria may well lead to a large number of newly diagnosed cases of diabetes. In its early stages,

Plasma Glucose	50-g Screening Test	100-g Diagnostic Test
TABLE 2-2 Screening and Diagnosis Scheme for Gestational Diabetes		
Fasting	—	95 mg/dl
1-h	140 mg/dl	180 mg/dl
2-h	—	155 mg/dl
3-h	—	140 mg/dl

(Adapted from American Diabetes Association,[2,7] with permission.)

type 2 diabetes can often be effectively treated with a healthy diet and regular physical activity.[1] (See Chapter 5.)

■ References

1. American Diabetes Association. Diabetes Info: New Recommendations to Lower the Diabetes Diagnosis Point. 1997. Available at: http://www.diabetes.org/ada/nwclass.html.
2. American Diabetes Association. Clinical Practice Recommendations 1998. Report of the Expert Committee on the diagnosis and classification of diabetes mellitus. *Diabetes Care*. 1998;21(suppl 1):S5–S19.
3. American Diabetes Association. Clinical Practice Recommendations 2000. Report of the Expert Committee on the diagnosis and classification of diabetes mellitus. *Diabetes Care*. 2000;23(suppl 1):S4–S19.
4. National Institute of Diabetes and Digestive and Kidney Diseases (NIDDK). Protocol for the Diabetes Prevention Program (DPP). Available at: http://www.niddk.nih.gov/patient/DPP/execsum.htm. Accessed on November 11, 2000.
5. Palmer P, Lernmark Å. Pathophysiology of type 1 (insulin-dependent) diabetes. In: Porte D Jr, Sherwin RS, eds. *Ellenberg & Rifkin's Diabetes Mellitus*. 5th ed. New York, NY: McGraw–Hill; 1997:455–486.
6. American Diabetes Association. Clinical Practice Recommendations 2000. Screening for type 2 diabetes. *Diabetes Care*. 2000;23(suppl 1):S20–S23.
7. American Diabetes Association. Clinical Practice Recommendations 2000. Gestational diabetes mellitus. *Diabetes Care*. 2000;23(suppl 1):S77–S79.

CHAPTER THREE

Complications of Diabetes: Assessing the Patient

Diabetes is a complex disease requiring continuing medical assessment and care to prevent acute complications and reduce the risk of long-term consequences. A primary purpose of patient assessment is to determine the existence and degree of diabetes complications. The Diabetes Control and Complications Trial (DCCT) followed the effects of intensive glucose control on young—average age, 27 years—type 1 individuals. These patients were divided into primary prevention (1- to 5-year diagnosis of diabetes) and secondary intervention (a diagnosis of 1 to 15 years) cohorts. Published in 1993, the DCCT results showed that lowering blood glucose in type 1 diabetes unequivocally delays the onset and progression of microvascular complications.[1]

In 1977, researchers from Oxford University began the United Kingdom Prospective Diabetes Study (UKPDS), involving over 5,000 people with type 2 diabetes, to understand the best way to manage the disease and to prevent or delay serious complications. The average age of these patients was 53 years, and they were divided into groups receiving "intensive" and "conventional" treatment to determine the effects of intensive blood glucose control on the risk of complications of diabetes. For the 1,138 patients assigned to conventional treatment, the goal was to maintain a fasting plasma glucose (FPG) of < 270 mg/dl, whereas the 2,729 patients in the intensive treatment group had an FPG goal of 108 mg/dl.[2] Data published in 1998 showed that intensive control of blood glucose can significantly reduce nephropathy, retinopathy, and possibly neuropathy—results that have serious implications for the way patients are managed.[2,3] There is substantial evidence that glycemic control can delay or prevent the onset of complications; it is, therefore, the primary goal of diabetes management.

A medical history, physical examination, and laboratory tests are all essential components of the patient assessment process and are discussed later in this chapter. As shown in Chapter 4, practical lifestyle changes and pharmacologic interventions can be directed at patients with a high risk of complications.

■ Microvascular Complications

The progression of diabetic vascular disease is related to a combination of metabolic, hormonal, and genetic factors.[4] The specific vascular tissue affected and the stage of disease progression also have an impact on the development of complications.[4] Microvascular abnormalities are a systemic disease in diabetes. Diabetic microangiopathy leads to retinopathy, neuropathy, and renal dysfunction.[4]

RETINOPATHY

Diabetic retinopathy is the most frequent cause of new cases of blindness among adults between the ages of 20 and 74 years. Between 12,000 and 24,000 new cases of blindness due to diabetic retinopathy occur each year.[5] It is the most common eye disease related to diabetes and is twice as likely as cataracts and glaucoma to occur among people with diabetes.

Retinopathy is a highly specific vascular complication of both type 1 and type 2 diabetes, with a prevalence strongly related to the duration of the illness. Nearly all patients with type 1 diabetes have some degree of retinopathy after 20 years, as do more than 60% of those with type 2 diabetes.[6] Moreover, in up to 21% of individuals with type 2 diabetes, retinopathy is found at the time of diagnosis.[6]

Data strongly support the association of retinopathy with poor glucose control. The UKPDS and DCCT conclusively demonstrated that, although intensive therapy will not completely prevent retinopathy, improving blood glucose control in patients with type 1 or type 2 diabetes reduces the risk of developing retinopathy and slows the progression of the disease.[1] Moreover, the DCCT showed that the shorter the duration of type 1 diabetes before beginning intensive therapy, the better the results. In this study, mean HbA_{1c} was the predominant predictor of retinopathy progression.[7]

In the DCCT, patients in the primary prevention group had no retinopathy when they entered the study, whereas patients in the secondary intervention group had very mild to moderate nonproliferative retinopathy.[1] After 6 years of follow-up monitoring, the primary prevention group undergoing intensive treatment had a 76% reduction in the adjusted mean risk of retinopathy. The secondary intervention cohort receiving intensive treatment had a 54% decrease in the risk of disease progression.[1]

The UKPDS also showed significant reduction in the risk of microvascular complications. In this study, 36% of patients in each of the intensive and conventional treatment groups had retinopathy when they entered the study,[2] but a 21% decrease in the relative risk of retinopathy was seen at the 12-year follow-up assessment in the group receiving intensive glucose management. At this time point, 49% of patients in the conventional group had retinopathy, a statistically significant difference from the 39% of patients with retinopathy in the intensive group.

NEPHROPATHY

The ADA reports that each year in the United States more than 20,000 people with diabetes are diagnosed with end-stage renal disease (ESRD), the final stage of nephropathy. Although most people with diabetes do not develop nephropathy severe enough to cause kidney failure, diabetes is the most common cause of ESRD, accounting for about 40% of the new cases.[5] In 1995, more than 98,000 individuals with diabetes underwent dialysis or kidney transplantation.[5] African Americans and Native Americans develop nephropathy and ESRD at rates higher than the average, a poorly understood phenomenon.

Microalbuminuria is the earliest clinical sign of nephropathy (> 30 mg/day or 20 µg/min). In 80% of individuals with type 1 diabetes who develop sustained microalbuminuria and do not receive specific interventions, an increase in urinary albumin excretion of about 10–20% each year is seen until the development of clinical albuminuria ($\geq$ 300 mg/24 h or 200 µg/min) or overt nephropathy. This occurs over a period of 10 to 15 years. ESRD develops in 50% of type 1 diabetes patients with overt nephropathy within 10 years and in > 75% by 20 years. Generally, the prevalence of microalbuminuria and overt nephropathy observed shortly after diagnosis is higher in patients with type 2 diabetes than in those with type 1, because type 2 diabetes is often present for many years before it is diagnosed. Microalbuminuria progresses to overt nephropathy in 20–40% of patients with type 2 diabetes when specific interventions are not provided. By 20 years, the disease in 20% of patients with type 2 diabetes will have progressed to ESRD. However, because this group has a greater risk of death from coronary artery disease (CAD), more cases of advanced nephropathy leading to ESRD may not be observed.[8]

In the DCCT primary prevention cohort, patients with type 1 diabetes had urinary albumin excretion < 40 mg/24 h; in the secondary intervention group, all patients had urinary albumin excretion < 200 mg/24 h.[1] With intensive glucose management, the mean adjusted risk of microalbuminuria ($\geq$ 40 mg/24 h) was reduced 34% in the primary prevention group and 43% in the secondary intervention group. The risk of albuminuria ($\geq$ 300 mg/24 h) was decreased 56% in the secondary intervention group.[1]

In the UKPDS trial, only 2% of patients who entered the study had proteinuria.[2] After 12 years of follow-up care, 10% in the conventional treatment group had signs of progressive disease, compared with 7% in the intensive glucose control group.[2] By year 12, a 33% reduction in the relative risk of microalbuminuria (> 50 mg/L) was seen in patients with intensive glucose control.[2]

As demonstrated by these results, intensive therapeutic intervention has the potential to improve a patient's quality of life by preserving kidney function and preventing or delaying ESRD, dialysis, and transplantation.

NEUROPATHY

Significant clinical neuropathy can develop within the first 10 years after diagnosis of diabetes; the longer a patient has diabetes, the higher is his or her risk of developing this pathology. Sixty percent of patients exhibit some form of neuropathy, but in 30–40% of patients there are no symptoms. Diabetic neuropathy appears more commonly among smokers, those over 40 years old, and people with uncontrolled diabetes. The mechanisms by which glucose control relates to complications are complex, yet studies have shown that glucose control may delay the progression or prevent the development of neuropathy.[9] For example, results of the DCCT research showed that intensive therapy for type 1 diabetes reduced the appearance of neuropathy at 5 years.[1]

In the UKPDS trial, 11% of patients had signs of neuropathy based on a biothesiometer reading of > 25 V.[2] Neuropathy as measured by absent reflexes did not differ between conventional and intensive glucose management groups, but at 15 years, the risk of neuropathy as measured by biothesiometer readings showed a 40% reduction in the intensive treatment group.[2]

Data presented by the DCCT on patients with type 1 diabetes showed that the appearance of neuropathy could be reduced. In the DCCT study, baseline clinical neuropathy was present in 2–5% of individuals in the primary prevention group and in 9% of those in the secondary intervention group.[1] The use of intensive therapy reduced the onset of neuropathy at 5 years by 69% in patients in the primary prevention cohort and by 57% in the secondary intervention cohort.[1] The study found that all components of the definition of neuropathy were reduced with intensive therapy: abnormal findings on neurologic examination, abnormal nerve conduction, and abnormal results on autonomic nerve testing.[1]

■ Cardiovascular Complications

Heart disease is the leading cause of diabetes-related death. Seventy-five to 80% of adults with diabetes die from coronary heart disease, cerebrovascular disease, or peripheral vascular diseases; this percentage is approximately two to four times higher than in adults without diabetes mellitus.[5] Postmortem studies from the 1950s and 1960s confirmed that people with diabetes exhibit an increased prevalence of CAD.[10–12]

The macrovascular complications of both type 1 and type 2 diabetes result from an acceleration of atherosclerosis and an increase in thrombosis.[4] Cardiovascular complications are two to six times more frequent than the microvascular complications of type 2 diabetes.[13] With type 2 diabetes, CAD appears to develop at a younger age, has a higher rate of diffuse multivessel heart disease, poor coronary vasodilatory reserve, worse outcome after the first myocardial infarction, and increased likelihood of developing congestive heart failure.[14]

In addition to assessing the risk of microvascular complications, the UKPDS examined the impact of intensive blood glucose and blood pressure control on macrovascular disease and found that the intensive control group had a 16% reduction in the risk of myocardial infarction. This reduction in risk approached statistical significance and suggests the benefits of tight control.[2]

LIPIDS

In patients with type 2 diabetes, the pattern of dyslipidemia typically consists of elevated triglycerides and decreased high-density lipoprotein (HDL) cholesterol. Low-density lipoprotein (LDL) cholesterol levels are usually not significantly different from those levels in individuals without diabetes; however, elevated non-HDL cholesterol (LDL plus very-low-density lipoprotein [VLDL]) may be seen. Individuals with type 2 diabetes usually have a tendency toward smaller, denser LDL particles, which may increase atherogenicity despite normal absolute LDL levels.[15] Higher blood triglycerides and lower HDL cholesterol are linked to the abnormal physiology produced by insulin resistance or inadequate insulin action. According to the ADA, an association among glucose and insulin levels, obesity, high triglyceride levels, and lower HDL cholesterol levels can be found in nearly all diabetic populations in the United States.[16] In addition, elevated serum lipids have been associated with hard exudates and visual loss.[6] Long-term treatment of lipid levels has been shown to improve survival rates in patients with heart disease.[17]

HYPERTENSION

It is estimated that 60–65% of individuals with diabetes have hypertension,[5] and hypertension in individuals with diabetes has been associated with the development of chronic complications. Patients with type 1 diabetes and persistent hypertension often develop nephropathy. In patients with type 2 diabetes, a syndrome involving hypertension with glucose intolerance, insulin resistance, dyslipidemia, obesity, and CAD is frequently seen. Hypertension is also a risk factor for macular edema and is associated with proliferative diabetic retinopathy.

The findings of the UKPDS trials confirmed the association between hypertension and the complications of type 2 diabetes and provided valuable information on the control of hypertension in this patient group. The UKPDS group found, in comparing a group of patients with tight blood pressure control (144/82 mm Hg) versus a less tight control (154/87 mm Hg), that significant reductions in the risk of macrovascular and microvascular complications occurred. Overall, a 24% reduction in the risk of developing any end-point condition related to diabetes was seen with tight control.[18] Additionally, there was a 32% reduction in risk of deaths related to diabetes, two thirds of which were cardiovascular; a 34% reduction in the risk of all macrovascular disease (myocardial infarction, sudden stroke, peripheral vascular disease [PVD]); and a 37% reduction in risk of microvascular disease.[18] Moreover, the risk of deterioration in retinopathy from baseline by two or more steps was reduced by 34% by 7.5 years. Furthermore, at 9 years, a 47% reduction in the risk of loss of vision by three or more lines in both eyes as measured by an Early Treatment Diabetic Retinopathy Study (ETDRS) chart was observed. At 6 years of follow-up monitoring, tight-control patients had a 29% reduction in the risk of urinary albumin concentration of ≥ 50 mg/L.[18] Consequently, tight blood pressure control in patients with type 2 diabetes and hypertension is key to reducing death related to diabetes and its clinical complications and in maintaining quality of life.

STROKE

Stroke is another vascular disease common in diabetes patients. Although the UKPDS did not show that tight glycemic control affects the risk of stroke, it did demonstrate the benefits of blood pressure control (144/82 mm Hg) in patients with type 2 diabetes. Improved blood pressure control resulted in a 44% reduction in the risk of fatal and nonfatal strokes.[18]

■ Medical History*

Among patients with unrecognized diabetes, the answers provided through a medical history will uncover symptoms that help establish a diagnosis. If a diagnosis of diabetes is suspected or has already been made, a medical history will confirm the diagnosis, involve a review of treatment, help determine the level of glycemic control, assess the presence (or absence) of complications, and help the physician form a management plan and provide continuing care (see also Chapter 4). Medical history may be divided into the following categories:

GENERAL DIABETES

- Symptoms (Table 3-1), results of laboratory tests, and special examination results related to diabetes
- History of disease—age, symptoms, treatment since onset

---

* Adapted from American Diabetes Association,[20] with permission.

TABLE 3-1
Classic Diabetes Signs and Symptoms

Type 1	Type 2
High levels of sugar in the blood and urine	Same as type 1 plus:
Frequent urination (and/or bedwetting in children)	Blurred vision
Extreme hunger, thirst, or weight loss	Repeated or hard-to heal infections of the gums, skin, vagina, or bladder
Weakness, tiredness	
Feeling edgy, moody	Tingling or loss of feeling in hands and feet
Nausea, vomiting	Dry, itchy skin

- Prior HbA_{1c} test results
- Family history of diabetes and other endocrine disorders
- Lifestyle—cultural, psychosocial, educational, and economic factors that might influence diabetes management

DIET AND EXERCISE

- Eating patterns, nutritional status, and weight history; growth and development in children and adolescents
- Exercise history

DIABETES MANAGEMENT

- Details of previous treatment programs, including nutrition and diabetes self-management training
- Current treatment of diabetes, including medications, meal plan, results of glucose monitoring, and patient's use of the data

DIABETES COMPLICATIONS

- Frequency, severity, and cause of acute complications such as diabetic ketoacidosis (DKA) and hypoglycemia
- Symptoms and treatment of chronic complications associated with diabetes—eye, kidney, nerve, genitourinary (including sexual), bladder, gastrointestinal, heart, peripheral vascular, foot, and cerebrovascular
- Risk factors for atherosclerosis—smoking, hypertension, obesity, dyslipidemia, and family history

GENERAL MEDICAL

- Prior or current infections, particularly skin, foot, dental, and genitourinary
- History and treatment of other conditions, including endocrine and eating disorders
- Gestational history—hyperglycemia, delivery of an infant weighing > 9 lb, preeclampsia, stillbirth, polyhydramnios, or other complications of pregnancy
- Other medications that may affect blood glucose levels

■ Physical Examination*

In the physical examination, the signs to watch for include thyroid disease and infections. The former is especially important among patients with type 1 diabetes, who harbor an increased frequency of autoimmune disease. Poorly controlled diabetes creates a higher risk for infections; for children, it can mean delayed growth and maturation. In addition, although such a situation is very rare, be alert for

---

* Adapted from American Diabetes Association,[20] with permission.

signs of diseases that can cause secondary diabetes, such as hemo-chromatosis, pancreatic disease, and endocrine disorders such as acromegaly, pheochromocytoma, and Cushing's syndrome. The following are important factors to include in the physical examination:

GENERAL

- Height and weight measurement (and comparison with norms in children and adolescents)
- Sexual maturation staging (during peripubertal period)
- Abdominal examination (e.g., hepatomegaly)
- Thyroid palpation

MICROVASCULAR COMPLICATIONS

- Ophthalmoscopic examination, preferably with dilation, for signs of retinopathy
- Hand/finger and foot examination for signs of neuropathy (proprioception to sharp/dull)
- Neurologic examination (reflexes, motor strength)
- Skin examination for signs of diabetic dermopathy

MACROVASCULAR COMPLICATIONS

- Cardiac examination for signs of macrovascular disease (bruits, cardiomegaly, rales)
- Blood pressure determination (with orthostatic measurements, when indicated) and comparison with age-related norms
- Evaluation of pulses (by palpation and auscultation)

INFECTION

- Oral examination for signs of periodontal disease

- Skin examination for signs of slow-healing wounds, infection at sites of insulin injection

■ Laboratory Evaluation*

Blood glucose and urine ketone testing should be available in the office for immediate use as needed. In addition, each patient should undergo laboratory tests appropriate to the person's general medical condition. Certain tests should be conducted to establish the diagnosis of diabetes, determine the degree of glycemic control, and define associated complications and risk factors. These tests include the following:

GENERAL

- FPG; a random plasma glucose may be obtained in a symptomatic patient for establishing a diagnosis
- HbA$_{1c}$ test
- Thyroid function test(s), when indicated

MICROVASCULAR COMPLICATIONS

- Serum creatinine in adults; in children if proteinuria is present
- Urinalysis—glucose, ketones, protein, sediment
- Determination for microalbuminuria (e.g., timed specimen or the albumin-to-creatinine ratio in pubertal patients who have had diabetes at least 5 years, and in all patients with type 2 diabetes)
- Urine culture, if sediment is abnormal or symptoms are present

---

* Adapted from American Diabetes Association,[20] with permission.

MACROVASCULAR COMPLICATIONS

- Fasting lipid profile—total cholesterol, HDL cholesterol, triglycerides, LDL cholesterol (if triglycerides are consistently > 400 mg/dl, LDL cannot be calculated, and therefore a direct-measure LDL may be warranted)
- Electrocardiogram (in adults)
- Stress testing if indicated

◼ Conclusion

Analysis has shown that the greatest survival benefits to people with diabetes will come from the cessation of smoking and the correction of dyslipidemia and hypertension, combined with intensive glycemic control.[19] The correction of modifiable risk factors such as obesity, hypertension, smoking, and dyslipidemia should be included in medical management goals.

An annual examination for individuals with diabetes should ensure the early detection of diabetic complications. Vigilant assessment of the status of the disease and early detection of the complications are imperative to increasing the quality of life and the length of survival in individuals with diabetes.

◼ References

1. Diabetes Control and Complications Trial Research Group. The effect of intensive treatment of diabetes on the development and progression of long-term complications in insulin-dependent diabetes mellitus. *New Engl J Med.* 1993;329:977–986.
2. UK Prospective Diabetes Study (UKPDS) Group. Intensive blood-glucose control with sulphonylureas or insulin compared with conventional treatment

and risk of complications in patients with type 2 diabetes (UKPDS 33). *Lancet.* 1998;352:837–853.

3. American Diabetes Association. Clinical Practice Recommendations 2000. Implications of the United Kingdom Prospective Diabetes Study. *Diabetes Care.* 2000;23(suppl 1):S27–S31.

4. Feener EP, King GL. Vascular dysfunction in diabetes mellitus. *Lancet.* 1997;350(suppl I):9–13.

5. National Institute of Diabetes and Digestive and Kidney Diseases (NIDDK). Diabetes Statistics. NIH Publication No. 99-3892. March 1999. E-text posted September 1999. Available at: http://www.niddk.nih.gov/health/diabetes/pubs/dmstats/dmstats.htm. Accessed August 8, 2000.

6. American Diabetes Association. Clinical Practice Recommendations 2000. Diabetic retinopathy. *Diabetes Care.* 2000;23(suppl 1):S73–S76.

7. Diabetes Control and Complications Trial Research Group. The relationship of glycemic exposure (HbA$_{1c}$) to the risk of development and progression of retinopathy in the Diabetes Control and Complications Trial. *Diabetes.* 1995;44:968–983.

8. American Diabetes Association. Clinical Practice Recommendations 2000. Diabetic nephropathy. *Diabetes Care.* 2000;23(suppl 1):S69–S72.

9. National Institute of Diabetes and Digestive and Kidney Diseases (NIDDK). Diabetic Neuropathy: The Nerve Damage of Diabetes. NIH Publication No. 95-3185. July 1995. Updated November 27, 1996. Available at: http://www.niddk.nih.gov/DiabeticNeuropathy/DiabNeur.htm. Accessed August 11, 2000.

10. Goldberg S, Alex M, Blumenthal HT. Sequelae of arteriosclerosis of the aortic and coronary arteries: a statistical study in diabetes mellitus. *Diabetes.* 1958; 7:98–108.

11. Feldman M, Feldman J Jr. The association of coronary occlusion and infarction with diabetes mellitus: a necropsy study. *Am J Med Sci.* 1954;228:53–56.

12. Goodale F, Daoud AS, Florentine R, et al. Chemicoanatomic studies of arteriosclerosis and thrombosis in diabetics. I: coronary arterial wall thickness, thrombosis, and myocardial infarcts in autopsied North Americans. *Exp Mol Pathol.* 1962;1:353–363.

13. Meigs JB, Singer DE, Sullivan LM, et al. Metabolic control and prevalent cardiovascular disease in non-insulin-dependent diabetes mellitus (NIDDM): The NIDDM Patient Outcomes Research Team. *Am J Med.* 1997;102:38–47.

14. Nathan DM, Meigs J, Singer DE. The epidemiology of cardiovascular disease in type 2 diabetes mellitus: how sweet it is . . . or is it? *Lancet.* 1997;350 (suppl I):4–9.

15. American Diabetes Association. Clinical Practice Recommendations 2000. Management of dyslipidemia in adults with diabetes. *Diabetes Care.* 2000; 23(suppl 1):S57–S60.

16. American Diabetes Association. Consensus Statement: Detection and management of lipid disorders in diabetes. *Diabetes Care*. 1993;16:828–834.

17. Scandinavian Simvastatin Survival Study Group. Randomised trial of cholesterol lowering in 4444 patients with coronary heart disease: the Scandinavian Simvastatin Survival Study (4S). *Lancet*. 1994;344:1383–1389.

18. United Kingdom Prospective Diabetes Study Group. Tight blood pressure control and risk of macrovascular and microvascular complications in type 2 diabetes (UKPDS 38). *BMJ*. 1998;317:703–713.

19. Eastman RC, Keen H. The impact of cardiovascular disease on people with diabetes: the potential for prevention. *Lancet*. 1997;350(suppl I):29–32.

20. American Diabetes Association. Clinical Practice Recommendations 2000. Standards of medical care for patients with diabetes mellitus. *Diabetes Care*. 2000;23(suppl1):S32–S42.

CHAPTER FOUR

Management of Diabetes: Designing a Plan

For most patients, a diagnosis of diabetes means making a considerable adjustment in lifestyle, health care, and their way of thinking about themselves and their vulnerability to illness. The physician must work cooperatively with the patient to develop a realistic and manageable plan for lifelong treatment of diabetes. A management plan should be developed as a therapeutic alliance between the patient and physician. The plan should focus on the involvement of the patient in problem solving, behavior modification, and goal setting as much as possible. Patient self-management should be encouraged.

Key components of the management plan should include the following:

- Short- and long-term goals
- Medications
- Monitoring of glycemic status: use of self-monitored blood glucose (SMBG), urine ketones, and recordkeeping
- Medical nutritional therapy
- Lifestyle and behavioral changes, including smoking cessation and exercise recommendations
- Annual referral to an eye specialist and other specialty consultations as needed

- Agreement for continuing support and return appointments
- A process for managing acute problems
- Annual pneumococcal and influenza vaccines
- Discussion of contraception, issues of pregnancy, and preconception care for women of childbearing age
- Self-management training processes for patient and family[1]

As successful diabetes treatment depends on the knowledge and involvement of the patient, self-management education is the foundation of disease management. Self-management education or training is the process of providing a patient with the skills and information needed to perform self-care and improve glycemic control on a day-to-day basis. Each aspect of the management plan must be understood and agreed on by the patient for full participation. The ADA has developed standards for diabetes self-management programs. The content of such programs should be designed with consideration of specific characteristics of the target population, the type of diabetes, cultural influences, and learning ability.[2] Ideally, the patient education process is managed by a team of professionals with expertise in diabetes management.

■ The Team Approach

The team approach of managing diabetes encourages physicians to coordinate a team of professionals to oversee the care of diabetic patients. Ideally, the team should include the following group of health care–related professionals:

- Certified diabetes educator
- Registered dietitian
- Exercise physiologist

- School nurse and/or teachers for pediatric patients
- Pharmacist

Physicians may also need to refer patients to the following specialists:

- Endocrinologist
- Ophthalmologist
- Neurologist
- Cardiologist
- Podiatrist
- Dentist
- Urologist
- Dermatologist
- Social worker/therapist/psychiatrist/psychologist

It is also understood that most primary care providers may not have easy access to the health care professionals outlined above. However, readily available information and educational materials from Internet sources and resources such as the ADA and the Juvenile Diabetes Foundation (JDF) can address those needs.

It is important not to underestimate the need for psychological support, especially soon after diagnosis. Often patients and their families feel bewildered by the array of new terms, devices, and requirements of care. In some cases, patients feel so overwhelmed it affects their ability to manage their disease. Depression, which occurs in about 5% of the general population, strikes 15–20% of patients with diabetes. Studies have also linked depression with poor glucose control and poor compliance with diabetes treatment regimens. Antidepressants or cognitive therapy can help patients improve their outlook and maintain their blood glucose at acceptable levels.[3]

■ Specific Treatment Goals

TYPE 1 DIABETES

As discussed in Chapter 3, the DCCT showed unequivocally that lowering blood glucose in type 1 diabetes delays the onset and progression of retinopathy, nephropathy, and neuropathy by 50–75% when compared with conventional programs.[4] The goal of glycemic control in type 1 diabetes is to lower HbA_{1c} values to maximize prevention of complications. The following aspects of management are suggested to attain this goal:[1]

- SMBG at least three or four times each day
- Medical nutrition therapy
- Self-management training
- If needed, hospitalization for initiation of therapy

TYPE 2 DIABETES

The landmark UKPDS showed that intensive control of blood glucose can significantly reduce nephropathy, retinopathy, and possibly neuropathy in patients with type 2 diabetes. A 25% risk reduction in microvascular end points was seen with intensive blood glucose control[5,6] (see Chapter 3). These results suggest a multiple risk management approach to type 2 diabetes, which includes exercise, diet, weight reduction, medication, monitoring of glycemic status, and reduction of risk factors.[1] The ADA-recommended goals for glycemic control are listed in Table 4-1.

■ Medications

Results of a UKPDS study in which follow-up monitoring with type 2 diabetes patients was conducted for 9 years demonstrated that with time there is a predictable progressive decline in β-cell function and

Stage	Normal	Goal	Action Suggested
Whole blood values			
Average preprandial glucose (mg/dl)	< 100	80–120	< 80 or > 140
Average bedtime glucose (mg/dl)	< 110	100–140	< 100 or > 160
Plasma values			
Average preprandial glucose (mg/dl)	< 110	90–130	< 90 or > 150
Average bedtime glucose (mg/dl)	< 120	110–150	< 110 or > 180
HbA$_{1c}$ (%)	< 6	< 7	> 8

TABLE 4-1
Goals of Glycemic Control for Individuals with Diabetes

Note: Values are generalized to the entire population of individuals with diabetes. Those with comorbidity, the very young, elderly, and others with unusual circumstances may warrant other treatment goals. "Action suggested" may include additional education, change in medication, referral to an endocrinologist, change in SMBG, or increased physician monitoring. (Adapted from American Diabetes Association,[1] with permission.)

a resultant failure in glycemic control. This failure was seen with the use of monotherapy, including sulfonylureas, metformin, and insulin. The study concluded that within 3 years after diagnosis, 50% of patients will need combination pharmacologic therapy to achieve tight glycemic control and that by 9 years, approximately 75% of patients will need multiple therapies to achieve HbA$_{1c}$ levels below 7%. By 9 years, a majority of patients will need the incorporation of insulin therapy to their management plans to reach target blood glucose goals.[7] The ADA has developed a treatment algorithm for the management of patients with type 2 diabetes that reflects this progressive need for multiple therapies and insulin (Figure 4-1). Details about the use of oral antihyperglycemic medications can be found in Chapter 6 and of insulin in Chapter 7.

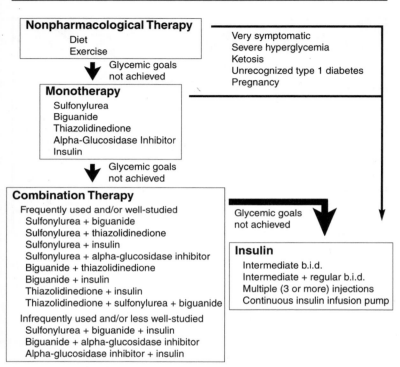

Figure 4-1. Algorithm for treatment of type 2 diabetes (Adapted from American Diabetes Association,[8] with permission.)

■ Monitoring

BLOOD GLUCOSE TESTING

In recent years, SMBG has revolutionized diabetes management. Diabetes educators are teaching an increasing number of patients how to monitor their own blood glucose levels in an effort to maintain tight control. All treatment programs developed for patients with type 1 diabetes should involve routine daily SMBG monitoring to optimize medication and prevent asymptomatic hypoglycemia. It is recommended that patients perform SMBG three to four times a day (Table 4-2). In individuals with type 2 diabetes, the frequency of testing depends on how well patients are maintaining glucose control. Table 4-2 offers a typical testing strategy.

Patients should also be encouraged to keep daily records that will be reviewed at physician visits (Figure 4-2). Glucose meters usually include a logbook; patients can also order such record sheets by mail (see Patient Resources). Physicians should instruct patients that many glucose meters store daily readings and can provide average glucose levels over time. In this way, physicians can determine whether patients are meeting their glycemic, diet, and exercise goals.

URINE TESTING

For patients who cannot perform SMBG, urine glucose testing may be considered. However, urine glucose testing provides only a

TABLE 4–2 Self-Monitored Blood Glucose Testing Frequency	
Patients with Type 1 Diabetes	Patients with Type 2 Diabetes
Before meals and at bedtime (some patients measure 2 hours after breakfast and dinner to monitor postprandial response)	Twice daily, if needed to achieve glycemic goals; vary the hour of testing to provide a more accurate assessment over time; patients taking insulin may need to check three or four times per day

Note: Routine laboratory blood glucose testing by health care providers should be used as follow-up assessment for SMBG.

Today's Date:

Foods and Beverages			Dietary Exchanges or Grams						
Breakfast Time:	Amount	Starch	Fruit	Milk	Veg	Meat	Fat	Free

Snack Time:	Amount	Starch	Fruit	Milk	Veg	Meat	Fat	Free

Lunch Time:	Amount	Starch	Fruit	Milk	Veg	Meat	Fat	Free

Snack Time:	Amount	Starch	Fruit	Milk	Veg	Meat	Fat	Free

Dinner Time:	Amount	Starch	Fruit	Milk	Veg	Meat	Fat	Free

Snack Time:	Amount	Starch	Fruit	Milk	Veg	Meat	Fat	Free

Medicines Insulin Supplements	Amount	Time	Time	Time	Time	Time	Time

BLOOD GLUCOSE MONITORING

Time	Level	Time	Level	Time	Level	Time	Level	Time	Level	Time	Level

KETONE MONITORING

Time	Level	Time	Level	Time	Level	Time	Level	Time	Level	Time	Level

PHYSICAL ACTIVITY AND EXERCISE

Activity	Intensity	Time Started	Duration

FOOT CARE AND CONDITION (inspection, cleansing, shoes, corns, infections, etc.)

_____

_____

COMMENTS (moods, stresses, food testing, medication changes, illness, triumphs, etc.)

_____

_____

_____

WEIGHT

Figure 4-2. Sample patient daily log. (From HealthLogs,[10] with permission.)

rough estimate of blood glucose levels and provides no information on blood glucose levels below 180 mg/dl, which is the renal threshold in most patients.[9]

Whereas urine glucose testing may not play a significant role in glucose management, urine ketone testing remains an important part of monitoring among patients with type 1 diabetes, patients with gestational diabetes, and pregnant patients with preexisting diabetes. Ketones in the urine can indicate impending or even established ketoacidosis, a condition requiring immediate medical attention. It should be noted that ketone readings may be false positive during fasting and in first morning urine of pregnant women.[9]

All patients should test their urine for ketones during the following situations:

- Acute illness or stress
- Consistently elevated blood glucose levels (> 300 mg/dl)[9]
- Pregnancy
- Presence of ketoacidosis symptoms, such as nausea, vomiting, or abdominal pain

GLYCATED PROTEIN TESTING

Measurement of glycated proteins, primarily glycated hemoglobin (i.e., HbA_{1c} or total glycated hemoglobin), provides a quantitative, reliable measure of glycemia over an extended period of time. Glycated hemoglobin levels can be assessed by several methodologies. The HbA_{1c} test measures a specific glycated hemoglobin species and is commonly measured by ion-exchange chromotography methods. However, a *total* glycated hemoglobin level is essentially a measure of all glycated hemoglobin species, including the HbA_{1c} level. As such, reports of total glycated hemoglobin levels are generally higher than those of HbA_{1c} levels. Therefore, it is important that the primary care provider know, when comparing tests from other clinics, which level is specifically reported. A single measurement can quantify average glycemia over weeks or months. This information complements SMBG, which provides information only on day-to-day management, whereas the glycated hemoglobin value accurately reflects the previous 2 to 3 months of glycemic control.[9] Results of the DCCT showed a direct relationship between HbA_{1c} values and the risk of chronic diabetes complications. The ADA recommends that all patients with diabetes be routinely tested for HbA_{1c} levels every 3 months.

Optimal use of HbA_{1c} testing requires standardization of the assay; thus, the HbA_{1c} assay method used must be certified as traceable to the DCCT reference method.[9]

In addition to the glycated hemoglobin test, other assays measure the amount of glucose attached to serum proteins that have shorter half-lives in the circulation compared to hemoglobin. One commercially available assay called fructosamine is a reflection of glycated serum proteins, primarily albumin. As such, it reflects glycemic control over the previous 1 to 2 weeks. This technology for assessing fructosamine has been recently made available for patient home use and provides another tool to aid the patient in achieving optimal glucose control. However, the use of once-a-week fructosamine testing should not take the place of daily monitoring but should complement regular glycated hemoglobin tests.[11]

■ Measuring Tools

Acquiring blood samples, sometimes four or more times a day, can be painful and difficult for patients. Until noninvasive techniques (see Chapter 9) are widely available, the finger stick and blood glucose meter represent the state of the art in testing techniques.

Most glucose meters calculate blood glucose either chemically, by using an enzyme that changes color in the presence of glucose, or electrically, by measuring the current generated by glucose oxidation. In both cases, the patient places a drop of blood on a test strip for the meter to read. Some meters record up to 250 readings in memory, obviating the need for written logs. The most sophisticated systems include alarm clocks and record time, date, insulin doses, exercise, and food intake (including grams of carbohydrates eaten). In addition, computer programs are available that allow patients to analyze these data and obtain printouts showing trends in glucose control.

GLUCOSE METERS

Patients should adhere to the following procedures when using glucose meters:

- Because test strips can vary from lot to lot, calibrate them to the meter.
- Use only fresh strips that have not expired or changed color owing to chemical spoilage.
- Periodically calibrate the meter with a control solution.
- Keep the meter clean and free of dust, lint, and blood.
- Periodically compare meter readings to laboratory results during an office visit or session with a diabetes educator; the results should be within 15% of each other.
- Replace meter batteries regularly.
- Use smaller pen- or card-size meters for convenience and travel.

GLUCOSE STRIPS

When patients cannot use a blood glucose meter, they can always use visually read blood or urine strips as a backup measure. To read the strips, patients should note and do the following:

- Color patches usually graduate in increments of 20–30 mg/dl.
- To estimate glucose level, match the color of the test strip to the chart on the side of the vial; keep in mind that a patient may be color blind.
- Urine test strips are not specific as to the time or degree of glucose elevation in the blood.
- Do *not* make diabetes management decisions on the basis of urine readings.

KETONE STRIPS

Patients should note the following about ketone strips:

- Depending on manufacturer, ketone strips vary in the time they take to yield results, from 15 seconds to 2 minutes.
- Tests that use nitroprusside-containing reagents can yield false positive results when sulfhydryl drugs such as captopril are present.
- Acidic urine, due to agents such as ascorbic acid, may provide false negative results.
- Test strips exposed to air for long periods of time may give false negative results.
- Currently available urine ketone tests are not reliable for diagnosing or monitoring treatment of ketoacidosis. (Recently available methods that quantify β-hydroxybutyric acid have been found to be reliable, but are not available for home testing.[9])

LANCET FINGER STICKS

Patients should be aware of the following:

- Lancets are meant for one-time, one-person use only.
- Different lancets create different size blood drops; it is important to use the correct size for the test strip.

- Finger-sticking devices often feature two different caps to control the depth of poke; it is best to use the shallowest depth possible.
- Automatic lancing devices can be used by patients with limited dexterity.
- Some glucose meters feature a built-in lancet; replacement lancets must be designed to fit that machine.

■ Testing and Treating Diabetes at Special Times

DURING ILLNESS AND STRESS

Illness and stress can raise blood glucose, so physicians need to instruct patients that when they are experiencing stress or illness they should:

- Test blood glucose and ketones more frequently and record results
- Contact the physician about adjusting medication if they are unable to eat (especially in the presence of ketosis)
- Drink plenty of fluids
- Test urine for ketones if blood glucose is over 240 mg/dl or if vomiting or weight loss occurs
- Contact the physician immediately if any of the following exist:

    Persistent hyperglycemia (e.g., two sequential tests showing blood glucose > 300 mg/dl)

    Ketonuria

    Vomiting or diarrhea

    Mental clouding

    Respiratory difficulty

    Evidence of infection

DURING SCHOOL OR WORK ROUTINES

At school or at work, patients with diabetes can face different obstacles. Physicians need to reinforce the following points with their patients:

- Try to eat meals at the same time each day.
- Take medicine and test blood glucose as usual.
- Advise teachers, friends, or close coworkers of the signs of low blood glucose.
- Keep sugar-containing snacks on hand.
- Inform company or school medical personnel of the presence of diabetes.

DURING TRAVEL

Though patients may travel, they get no vacation from diabetes. Remind patients to do the following:

- Follow meal plans as much as possible when dining out; always carry a snack in case there is a wait to be served.
- Limit alcohol intake; if opting to drink, eat food when drinking and choose drinks made with club or sugar-free soda.
- On long car trips, drive early in the day; keep snacks in the car in case of hypoglycemia. If you have not eaten in a while, test your blood glucose before driving.
- When making air travel arrangements, request a special diabetic meal; carry snacks in case of delays.
- Never put medicines in a checked suitcase; always have direct access to insulin, insulin syringes, oral antihyperglycemic agents, and blood testing supplies.
- Carry extra supplies, a written prescription, and the name of a physician located at the destination.

- Carry medicine in special insulated bags to keep it from freezing or getting too hot.
- Carry a statement from the physician verifying your diabetes and need for insulin and syringes; always wear a medical alert tag.
- When crossing time zones, maintain eating and insulin schedules according to your internal clock for a day before switching to local time.

DURING PREGNANCY

During pregnancy, hyperglycemia can harm both mother and unborn baby. Thus, patients should bear the following in mind:

- Before and during pregnancy, keep glucose levels in normal range using daily SMBG.
- During pregnancy, insulin needs may change. Pregnant women may need to take more insulin and test blood glucose more often.
- Insulin has been shown to reduce fetal morbidity when added to medical nutritional therapy.
- Oral glucose-lowering agents are not recommended during pregnancy.[12]

HYPOGLYCEMIA

Hypoglycemia results from an excess of insulin in the blood, leading to excessively low levels of blood glucose. When it occurs, it is most often a side effect of insulin or sulfonylurea therapy, although it can also occur with other antihyperglycemic agents or after exercise.[13] Patients who appropriately monitor their glucose levels reduce their risk for hypoglycemia, but all patients should be alert to the signs outlined on page 51.

Hypoglycemic patients should be given foods containing carbohydrates or proteins to eat. Unconscious patients or patients with

---

Signs and Symptoms of Hypoglycemia

Adrenergic: weakness, palpitations, hunger, sweating, tremor, nausea (unusual), nervousness, irritability, vomiting (unusual), tachycardia, tingling (of mouth/fingers)

Neurologic: headache, confusion, visual disturbance, amnesia, hypothermia, seizures, mental dullness, coma

---

severe hypoglycemic reactions should be given parenteral glucagon or intravenous glucose. Family members or close associates should be taught how to administer parenteral glucagon in case of an emergency.

HYPERGLYCEMIA AND DIABETIC KETOACIDOSIS (DKA)

Every effort should be made to aggressively recognize and treat the early signs leading to DKA. Patients should notify their physician at the first signs of illness, such as nausea, vomiting, fever, or persistent hyperglycemia or ketonuria. These conditions require immediate attention and treatment. If the early signs leading to DKA are recognized, the physician can suggest more frequent injections of short-acting insulin and an increase in oral fluid intake to attempt to prevent progression to later stages of DKA and to restore metabolic balance. Clinical DKA is indicated by a blood glucose level of > 250 mg/dl, an arterial pH of < 7.2, plasma bicarbonate of ≤ 15 mEq/L, and ketones in the blood and urine. It is a life-threatening emergency requiring the following immediate treatment:

- Fluid replacement (isotonic saline or lactated Ringer's as initial solution)
- Insulin therapy (preferably intravenous)
- Potassium replacement

Signs and Symptoms of Hyperglycemia and Diabetic Ketoacidosis			
Polyuria	Polydipsia	Weakness	Hyperventilation
Dehydration	Anorexia	Blurred vision	Nausea
Vomiting	Abdominal pain		

- Exploration and treatment of possible precipitating events (e.g., infection, vascular events, medications)

Routine administration of bicarbonate is not recommended for most patients with DKA as it has not been associated with improved mortality or an accelerated clinical recovery and may actually complicate the clinical course in certain situations. Bicarbonate therapy is generally reserved for severe cases (i.e., pH ≤ 7.0).

It can take as long as a week after the patient is eating solid food to correct all the biochemical abnormalities associated with DKA. To prevent serious electrolyte imbalance and fluid overload, the patient's laboratory values should be monitored frequently. Glucose levels usually normalize more quickly than acidosis. Prematurely discontinuing or markedly decreasing insulin may aggravate ketoacidosis. Therefore, for hospitalized patients, supplemental insulin with glucose-containing solutions (D_5W) should be considered when the blood glucose concentration is < 300 mg/dl. This strategy allows the provider to continue insulin as it is needed to suppress ketogenesis, while minimizing the potential for hypoglycemia.

■ Continuing Care

Follow-up care is essential to managing patients with diabetes. The health care team needs to evaluate the patient's progress in

Components of the Continuing Care Visit

I. Contact frequency
   A. Daily for initiation of insulin or change in regimen
   B. Weekly for initiation of oral glucose-lowering agent(s) or change in regimen
   C. Routine diabetes visits
      1. Quarterly for patients who are not meeting goals
      2. Semiannually for other patients
II. Medical history
   A. Assess treatment regimen
      1. Frequency/severity of hypo-/hyperglycemia
      2. SMBG results
      3. Patient regimen adjustments
      4. Adherence problems
      5. Lifestyle changes
      6. Symptoms of complications
      7. Other medical illnesses
      8. Medications
      9. Psychosocial issues
III. Physical examination
   A. Physical examination annually
   B. Dilated eye examination annually
   C. Every regular diabetes visit
      1. Weight
      2. Blood pressure
      3. Previous abnormalities on the physical examination
      4. Foot examination
IV. Laboratory evaluation
   A. HbA$_{1c}$ assessed every 3–4 months
   B. Fasting plasma glucose (optional)
   C. Fasting lipid profile annually; if on lipid treatment, follow-up profiles as needed and monitor progress toward target goal
   D. Urinalysis for protein annually
   E. Microalbumin measurement annually (if urinalysis is negative for protein)
V. Review of management plan

A. Evaluate each visit
1. Short- and long-term goals
2. Glycemia
3. Frequency/severity of hypoglycemia
4. SMBG results
5. Complications
6. Control of dyslipidemia
7. Blood pressure
8. Weight
9. Medical nutrition therapy
10. Exercise regimen
11. Adherence with self-management training
12. Follow-up of referrals
13. Psychosocial adjustment
B. Evaluate annually
1. Knowledge of diabetes
2. Self-management skill

(Modified from American Diabetes Association,[14] with permission.)

attaining treatment goals and review any problems that have occurred.

■ References

1. American Diabetes Association. Clinical Practice Recommendations 2000. Standards of medical care for patients with diabetes mellitus. *Diabetes Care*. 2000;23(suppl 1):S32–S42.
2. American Diabetes Association. Clinical Practice Recommendations 1998. National standards for diabetes self-management education programs and American Diabetes Association review criteria. *Diabetes Care*. 1998;21(suppl 1):S95.
3. Lustman PJ, Griffith LS, Clouse RE, et al. Effects of nortriptyline on depression and glycemic control in diabetes: results of a double-blind placebo-controlled trial. *Psychosom Med*. 1997;59:241–250.

4. Diabetes Control and Complications Trial Research Group. The effect of intensive treatment of diabetes on the development and progression of long-term complications in insulin-dependent diabetes mellitus. *N Engl J Med.* 1993;329:977–986.

5. UK Prospective Diabetes Study (UKPDS) Group. Intensive blood-glucose control with sulphonylureas or insulin compared with conventional treatment and risk of complications in patients with type 2 diabetes (UKPDS 33). *Lancet.* 1998;352:837–853.

6. American Diabetes Association. Clinical Practice Recommendations 2000. Implications of the United Kingdom Prospective Diabetes Study. *Diabetes Care.* 2000;23(suppl 1):S27–S31.

7. Turner RC, Cull CA, Frighi V, Holman RR. Glycemic control with diet, sulfonylurea, metformin or insulin in patients with type 2 diabetes mellitus: progressive requirement for multiple therapies (UKPDS) 49). UK Prospective Diabetes Study Group. *JAMA.* 1999;281:2005–2012.

8. American Diabetes Association. Consensus Statement. The pharmacological treatment of hyperglycemia in NIDDM. *Diabetes Care.* 1995;18:1510–1518.

9. American Diabetes Association. Clinical Practice Recommendations 2000. Tests of glycemia in diabetes. *Diabetes Care.* 2000;23(suppl 1):S80–S82.

10. HealthLogs: Comprehensive Logbooks for Diabetics. Boise, ID: Dena E. Duncan, 1996.

11. Joslin Diabetes Center. Home fructosamine test. Available at http://www.joslin.harvard.edu/education/library/fructosamine_test.html. Accessed August 9, 2000.

12. American Diabetes Association. Clinical Practice Recommendations 2000. Gestational diabetes mellitus. *Diabetes Care.* 2000;23(suppl 1):S77–S79.

13. American Diabetes Association. Clinical Practice Recommendations 2000. Hypoglycemia and employment/licensure. *Diabetes Care.* 2000;23(suppl 1):S109.

14. American Diabetes Association. Clinical Practice Recommendations 1998. Standards of medical care for patients with diabetes mellitus. *Diabetes Care.* 1998;21(suppl 1):S23–S31.

CHAPTER FIVE

Guidelines for Diet and Exercise

People with diabetes must eat a well-balanced diet and exercise regularly to control their levels of glucose and decrease their need for medication (insulin and/or oral hypoglycemic agents). Proper diet and exercise can control type 2 diabetes in many cases and is postulated to delay its onset, improve cardiovascular health, and reduce insulin resistance. Because the diet and exercise recommendations for people with diabetes so closely match those for the general population, your patient need not feel singled out. His or her entire family can practice good health habits, giving them an opportunity to support the patient's needs.

■ Diet

Medical nutrition therapy is integral to successful diabetes management. Adhering to nutrition and meal planning is also one of the most challenging aspects of diabetes self-management.[1] There is no longer one "diabetic" or "ADA" diet. A recommended diet for a patient with diabetes is now based on individual assessment, treatment goals, and desired outcomes.[1]

A nutritional assessment is used to determine a nutrition prescription. The assessment is based on monitoring of glucose, glycated hemoglobin, lipids, blood pressure, renal status, weight, treatment goals, and individual patient lifestyle and ability. Sensitivity to cultural, ethnic, and financial factors is also important to facilitate patient self-management.[1]

Goals of Medical Nutrition Therapy

- Assist patient to make changes in nutrition to improve metabolic control
- Balance food intake, glucose-lowering pharmacotherapy, and physical activity level
- Achieve optimal lipid levels
- Attain and maintain optimal weight[1]
- Treat and prevent acute complications (such as hypoglycemia) and long-term complications (such as hypertension, cardiovascular disease (CVD), renal disease, and neuropathy)
- Improve overall health[1]

A coordinated effort by a team that includes the patient is required for success. A registered dietitian knowledgeable in implementing medical nutrition is a valuable asset to diabetes care.[1]

Once a year, patients should consult a dietitian to help plan, review, and revise a course of sound nutrition. The American Dietetic Association can provide a list of qualified local dietitians. (See Appendix 1.)

The best approach to nutrition, and the one most easily grasped by patients, is to use the Food Guide Pyramid, which was developed by the US Department of Agriculture, as a diet guide (Figure 5-1).

DAILY REGIMEN FOR PATIENTS USING INSULIN

The patient's usual food intake should be used as the basis for integrating insulin therapy into eating and exercise patterns. Physicians should instruct patients who self-administer insulin to institute the following procedures in their daily dietary regimens:

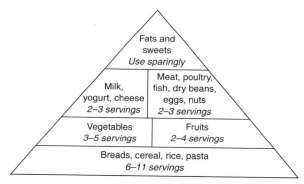

Figure 5-1. The Food Guide Pyramid.

- Synchronize meals with time-action of insulin preparation (see Chapter 7)
- Monitor blood glucose levels and adjust insulin doses for amount of food eaten
- Use multiple daily injections or an insulin pump for more flexibility in food intake

MEDICAL NUTRITION THERAPY FOR THE PATIENT WITH TYPE 2 DIABETES

The aim of nutritional therapy is to maintain glucose, blood pressure, and lipid goals. There is no evidence that supports eliminating any one food from the diet. Physicians should instruct patients to eat at consistent times, spacing meals throughout the day. Blood glucose levels, glycated hemoglobin, lipids, and blood pressure should be monitored at physician visits.

Traditional low-calorie diets are usually not effective in achieving long-term weight loss. Individuals with type 2 diabetes need to expand beyond weight loss to maintaining near-normal blood glucose levels. There is no one proven strategy for control. A nutritional meal plan with moderate calorie restriction (250 to 500 calories less than normal), reduction in total fat, and an increase in physical activity should be recommended. Increased sensitivity to insulin and improved blood glucose levels are associated with hypocaloric diets. A reduction in hyperglycemia, dyslipidemia, and hypertension have been seen with a moderate weight loss of 5 to 9 kg (around 11 to 20 lb).[1]

Physicians should instruct patients to derive ~10–20% of daily caloric intake from protein, both animal (lean meats) and vegetable (legume) sources, and to consult a dietitian about lowering protein intake to ~10% of calories with the onset of overt nephropathy. Once the glomerular filtration rate (GFR) begins to fall, restriction of protein to 0.6 g/kg/day should be considered.[1]

Diabetes is a strong independent risk factor for CVD; therefore, saturated fat should be restricted and cholesterol limited to < 300 mg/day.[1] Approximately 60–70% of caloric intake should be from monounsaturated fats and carbohydrates; the distribution of these calories may vary on the basis of therapy goals and individual assessment. Patients with normal weight and lipid levels should obtain < 30% of calories from fat, and < 10% of calories should be from saturated fats.[2]

Dietary fiber, which can be obtained from a wide variety of foods, is important. Patients should include 20 to 35 g of dietary fiber in their daily regimen. Although some soluble fibers may delay glucose absorption from the small intestine, the effect of dietary fiber on glycemic control is probably negligible. Restriction of sodium intake should be considered. Patients should limit their intake to 2,400 to 3,000 mg/day, less for those with mild to moderate hypertension. For patients with nephropathy and hypertension, ≤ 2,000 mg/day is recommended.

When diabetes is well controlled, *moderate use* of alcohol—no more than 2 drinks per day for men and no more than 1 drink per day for women—generally does not affect blood glucose. (One alcoholic beverage is equivalent to 12 oz beer, 5 oz wine, or 1.5 oz distilled spirits.) However, patients should note these precautions:

- Abstain from or reduce alcohol intake in the presence of pancreatitis, dyslipidemia, renal disease, or neuropathy.
- Because alcohol may increase the risk of hypoglycemia in those using insulin or sulfonylureas, such patients—if they choose to drink—should imbibe with a meal.
- Abstain from or reduce alcohol intake if weight control is at issue. Pregnant women and individuals with a history of alcohol abuse should also abstain from alcohol.

The signs of hypoglycemia can imitate the signs of drunkenness. If a person with diabetes experiences hypoglycemia after he or she is seen consuming alcohol, people may mistakenly assume he or she is inebriated when in fact the patient is suffering hypoglycemia. Physicians need to urge patients to drink in moderation, remain sober, and keep their wits about them. They may need to move quickly to self-administer treatment.

SWEETENERS

Sweeteners occur naturally or are sugars added to foods. Physicians should review the role of sweeteners in their patients' diets.

As part of a meal plan, *sucrose* does not impair blood glucose control in patients with type 1 or type 2 diabetes. Foods with high amounts of added sugars should be eaten sparingly. Although people with dyslipidemia should avoid large amounts of *fructose*, there is no reason to avoid fruits and vegetables, in which fructose occurs naturally, or moderate amounts of fructose-sweetened foods. There is no evidence that *nutritive sweeteners* such as corn syrup, fruit juice or fruit juice concentrate, honey, molasses, dextrose, or maltose offer any significant advantage or disadvantage over sucrose in terms of improving caloric content or glycemic response. *Sorbitol*, *mannitol*, and *xylitol* are common sugar alcohols that produce a lower glycemic response than sucrose and other carbohydrates. Although they offer no significant benefit, in large amounts they can create a laxative effect.

The US Food and Drug Administration (FDA) recently approved a new nonnutritive sweetener, sucralose, for use in food products. The new sweetener is made from table sugar and is 600 times as sweet as sugar. It cannot be digested; therefore, it adds no calories. Several studies have shown that the agent does not affect blood glucose levels.[3]

VITAMIN AND MINERAL SUPPLEMENTS

Physicians should discuss the following factors concerning vitamins and minerals with their patients[2]:

- Assuming adequate dietary intake, patients generally do not need supplements.

- Routine evaluation of serum *magnesium* levels is necessary because deficiency of this mineral can lead to insulin resistance, carbohydrate intolerance, and hypertension.

- In patients taking diuretics, *potassium* loss may warrant supplementation.

Some patients on long-term parenteral nutrition developed *chromium* deficiency, as noted in past studies, which was associated with glucose intolerance. Chromium replacement corrected the glucose abnormality, and chromium supplements are now routinely added to parenteral nutrition solutions. Significant beneficial effects of chromium have been demonstrated in recent studies. Improvements in altered glucose metabolism, ranging from mild glucose intolerance to overt diabetes, have been seen. A dose of 200 µg/day of chromium as chromium picolinate appeared to improve glucose and lipid variables in a study of type 2 diabetes in the Chinese population.[4] Women with gestational diabetes were observed to respond well to 4 to 8 µg/kg of chromium as chromium picolinate.[5] In addition, recent research has shown that corticosteroid therapy increases chromium loss and chromium supplementation can reverse steroid-induced diabetes.[6] Because of such recent and favorable observations using supplemental doses greater than those that have been used in the past, clinical research studies are ongoing and when completed may provide definitive recommendations for or against routine use of chromium supplementation in the management of diabetes.

■ Exercise

The potential benefits of exercise include improved glycemic control, weight loss, decreased risk of atherosclerosis, and stalled progression of metabolic abnormalities. Most improvement is due to increased insulin sensitivity.[7] With the right preparation and precautions, most people with diabetes can exercise safely—even take part in competitive sports, if they wish—and reap the benefits. If they are not already active, their disease provides a compelling reason to begin an exercise regimen and to stick with it. However, a person with diabetes should undergo a detailed medical evaluation before beginning an exercise program. The presence of macro- and microvascular complications that could be potentially worsened by exercise should be ruled out. Screening should focus on the following.

CARDIOVASCULAR STATUS

The patient's risk for CVD should be determined on the basis of the presence of risk factors[8]:

- Age > 35 years
- Type 2 diabetes > 10 years or type 1 diabetes > 15 years
- Presence of additional CVD risk factors, such as smoking
- Presence of microvascular disease
- Peripheral vascular disease
- Autonomic neuropathy

Patients with known coronary artery disease (CAD) should be evaluated for ischemic response to exercise, ischemic threshold, and risk of arrhythmia during exercise.[8]

RETINOPATHY

All patients with type 1 or type 2 diabetes should have annual dilated and comprehensive eye exams by an experienced ophthalmologist or optometrist. In patients with active proliferative retinopathy, strenuous exercise may precipitate vitreous hemorrhage or traction retinal detachment.[9] These patients should avoid weight-lifting, high-impact aerobic activities, and head-down positions.

NEPHROPATHY

Patients with overt nephropathy often have a reduced exercise capacity and self-limitation of activity. High-intensity exercise should be discouraged in this group.[8]

PERIPHERAL NEUROPATHY AND
PERIPHERAL ARTERIAL DISEASE (PAD)

Patients with diabetes should be assessed for peripheral arterial disease (PAD). Signs of intermittent claudication, decreased pulses, atrophy of subcutaneous tissue, cold feet, and hair loss should be evaluated. If peripheral neuropathy is found in the feet, limit weight-bearing and repetitive exercise. In patients with loss of protective sensation, the following exercises are contraindicated[8]:

- Jogging
- Prolonged walking
- Treadmill
- Step exercise

These patients should instead choose such exercises as cycling or swimming.

HYPERTENSION

Patients with hypertension should avoid weight-lifting or other activities that involve straining, such as isometric exercises.

AUTONOMIC NEUROPATHY

Autonomic neuropathy can limit exercise capacity and increase the risk of an adverse cardiovascular event during exercise. Resting tachycardia, orthostasis, or disturbances involving pupils, skin, or gastrointestinal or genitourinary systems may indicate cardiac autonomic neuropathy. The use of resting or stress thallium myocardial scintigraphy may be appropriate for ruling out the presence and extent of macrovascular CAD.[8]

ORGAN TRANSPLANTATION

When they are well enough, organ recipients should try aerobic and strength training because antirejection drugs can lead to weight gain and muscle wasting.

EXERCISE GUIDELINES FOR PATIENTS USING INSULIN

Physicians should instruct patients who self-administer insulin to include the following procedures before, during, and after exercise[10]:

- Always measure blood glucose before and after exercising.

- Do not begin exercise if blood glucose is very high (> 250 mg/dl) and if ketosis is present or if blood glucose is > 300 mg/dl without ketosis.

- If the blood glucose level is < 100 mg/dl, drink a cup of orange juice or eat a piece of fruit or bread and test 15 to 30 minutes later. Do not commence exercise until blood glucose rises above 100 mg/dl. (By testing twice before exercise, patients can determine whether their glucose level is stable or dropping.)

- Always begin exercise at least 1 hour after the last insulin injection. Avoid exercise during the time of peak insulin action. In the case of short-acting insulins, peak insulin action may be at 1 hour after injection; therefore, exercise should be delayed even longer.

- Note that insulin is absorbed much more quickly when injected close to muscles that are being exercised. The longer the interval between injecting insulin and exercising, the less important the injection site becomes.

- Eat something 2 to 3 hours before and after exercise.

- If hypoglycemic symptoms appear during exercise, *stop immediately* and measure glucose levels. (It might be wise for patients to exercise with a partner familiar with signs of low blood sugar in case the patient needs help. If going out alone, patients should wear diabetes identification tags and carry a cellular phone or money for a pay phone call.) However, given the acute onset of hypoglycemia, the patient may not have the luxury of time and therefore should always have a quick-acting carbohydrate source on hand during exercise (e.g., glucose tablets, raisins, or hard candy).

EXERCISE GUIDELINES FOR ALL PATIENTS WITH DIABETES

Physicians should inform patients that by keeping a log of blood glucose levels, medication taken, carbohydrates eaten, and duration and intensity of exercise, they will learn to gauge these variables and how they affect glycemic control. To prevent large swings in glucose levels, patients may need extra food for up to 24 hours after exercise, depending on duration and intensity of the workout.[10]

To prevent dehydration, patients need to drink plenty of water:

- 2 cups 2 hours before exercise
- 1 to 2 cups 30 minutes before exercise
- $\frac{1}{2}$ cup every 15 minutes during exercise

Additional instructions to patients should be the following[2]:

- Wear proper shoes and check your feet before and after exercise.
- Avoid exercise in extreme heat or cold and during periods of poor glycemic control.

IMPORTANT ELEMENTS OF EXERCISE

Patients with diabetes can benefit from aerobic activity, strength training, or both. In either case, a balanced exercise routine includes a warm-up of 5 to 10 minutes, at least 20 to 30 minutes of movement at the target heart rate, and a cool-down lasting until the heart rate has returned to normal. Stretching is another essential component of exercise and should be done while muscles are warm (after the warm-up and as part of the cool-down).[10] Specifics of these recommendations are outlined below. Physicians should use this information as a checklist when discussing exercise with patients.

Warm-Up

- Walk at a comfortable pace for 5 to 10 minutes.
- Stretch gently without bouncing or straining; yoga can help increase flexibility.
- Continue walking, slowly picking up the pace.

Aerobic Activity

Physicians should instruct patients to keep moving for 20 to 30 minutes. (Patients may have to work up to this gradually.) Whatever activity the patient chooses, he or she should be able to carry on a conversation during exercise without feeling out of breath. Ideally, patients should aim for a target heart rate, using the following formula[9]:

- Measure resting heart rate (HR_{rest}) first thing in the morning; count the number of beats in 1 minute.
- Determine maximum heart rate (HR_{max}) by subtracting your age from 220.
- Subtract HR_{rest} from HR_{max} to determine maximum heart rate reserve ($HR_{max\ reserve}$).
- Multiply $HR_{max\ reserve}$ by 0.5 and 0.7 to determine the range of heart rate reserve (i.e., 50–70% of maximum heart rate); when added to HR_{rest}, this yields the target range for an aerobic workout.

Strength Training[10]

- Certain patients should avoid weight-lifting (see above).
- Begin slowly and with lighter weights.
- Aim for increased strength and endurance for everyday activities.

- To increase endurance, choose a weight you can lift 15 to 20 times; rest and repeat the set 3 times.
- To increase strength and endurance, do the following:

    Use a weight you can lift 8 to 12 times; rest and repeat the set 3 times. Even at rest, larger muscles burn more calories, an aid to weight maintenance and better glucose control.

    Remember to warm up before and cool down after strength training.

    Exercise with a trainer, if possible, or at a gym that can provide assistance.

    Allow a day off between sessions or alternate upper and lower body training.

Cool-Down

- Keep moving, but at an easier pace, until heart rate returns to normal.
- Stretch muscles while still warm.
- Do not put the head below the level of the heart until cool-down is complete.

STAYING MOTIVATED

Physicians need to encourage their patients to remain motivated and to continue with their exercise programs. Patients should:

- Think of exercise as part of a daily routine
- To prevent boredom, vary the routine: alternate aerobic exercise on one day with strength training the next
- Choose activities they enjoy
- Work out with a partner for safety, companionship, and encouragement

- Set realistic goals
- Reward themselves (e.g., a new pair of running shorts or a soak in the hot tub)
- Take note of progress: when clothes fit better, energy level increases, glycemic control improves

■ References

1. American Diabetes Association. Clinical Practice Recommendations 2000. Nutritional recommendations and principles for people with diabetes mellitus. *Diabetes Care*. 2000;23(suppl 1):S43–S46.

2. American Diabetes Association. Clinical Practice Recommendations 1998. Nutrition recommendations and principles for people with diabetes mellitus. *Diabetes Care*. 1998;21(suppl 1):S32–S35.

3. FDA Consumer page. Sugar substitutes: Americans opt for sweetness and lite. Food and Drug Administration Web site. Available at: http://cfsan.fda.gov/~dms/fdsugar.html. Accessed July 26, 2000.

4. Anderson RA, Cheng N, Bryden NA, et al. Elevated intakes of supplemental chromium improve glucose and insulin variables in individuals with type 2 diabetes. *Diabetes*. 1997;46:1786–1791.

5. Jovanovic-Peterson L, Guitierrez M, Peterson C. Chromium supplementation for gestational diabetic women (GDM) improves glucose tolerance and decreases hyperinsulinemia. *Diabetes*. 1996;45(suppl 2):337A.

6. Ravina A, Slezak L, Mirsky N, Bryden NA, Anderson RA. Reversal of corticosteroid-induced diabetes mellitis with supplemental chromium. *Diabetic Medicine*. 1999;16:164–167.

7. Bloomgarden ZT. American Diabetes Association annual meeting, 1998: Insulin resistance, exercise and obesity. *Diabetes Care*. 1999;22:517–522.

8. American Diabetes Association. Clinical Practice Recommendations 2000. Diabetes mellitus and exercise. *Diabetes Care*. 2000;23(suppl 1):S50–S54.

9. American Diabetes Association. Clinical Practice Recommendations 2000. Diabetic retinopathy. *Diabetes Care*. 2000;23(suppl 1):S73–S76.

10. Kelley DB, ed-in-chief. *American Diabetes Association Complete Guide to Diabetes*. Alexandria, Va: American Diabetes Association, 1996.

Oral Hypoglycemic Agents for the Treatment of Type 2 Diabetes Mellitus

Effective treatment for patients with type 2 diabetes is critically important for avoiding long-term complications of this disease, including retinopathy, nephropathy, and cardiovascular disease. The results of the Diabetes Control and Complications Trial (DCCT) demonstrate that tight glucose control delays the onset and slows the progression of diabetic retinopathy, nephropathy, and neuropathy in patients with type 1 diabetes mellitus.[1] The landmark United Kingdom Prospective Diabetes Study (UKPDS), published in 1998, was the largest study ever done in patients with type 2 dibetes. A major objective of the study was to compare the effects of either insulin or sulfonylurea drugs versus conventional (i.e., nutritional) therapy on intensive blood glucose control and to assess the risk of complications in this patient population.[2] The main, randomized group of the study included 3,867 newly diagnosed patients. The patients followed an initial 3-month dietary program and then were randomly assigned to intensive therapy with a sulfonylurea (either chlorpropamide, glibenclamide, or glipizide) or to insulin or conventional diet therapy. The goal of the intensive treatment group was to attain a fasting plasma glucose (FPG) < 6 mmol/l (180 mg/dl), and the aim of the conventional group was to maintain an FPG < 15 mmol/l (270 mg/dl). Metformin or insulin was added to the sulfonylureas when marked hyperglycemia was seen.[2] The median follow-up of the study was 10 years. During that time, the median HbA_{1c} values were significantly lower in the intensive therapy group than in the conventional arm (7.0% versus 7.9%),[2] and a 25% risk reduction in microvascular end points was seen in the intensive group compared to the result in conventional therapy.[2] Evidence of a 16% reduction in the risk of myocardial infarctions was also seen; although statistically significant differences in macrovascular complications were not noted, the data approached significance.[2]

In a secondary analysis, the UKPDS compared the effects of intensive glucose control on overweight patients: 342 were allocated to treatment with metformin, 951 were given chlorpropamide, glibenclamide, or insulin, and 411 received conventional diet therapy. The median HbA_{1c} value for the metformin group was 7.4% compared to 8.0% for the conventional therapy group. Compared to those on conventional therapy, metformin patients had a 32% lower risk for any diabetes-related end point, a 39% lower risk for myocardial infarction, and a 30% reduction in all macrovascular disease.[3] Although metformin demonstrated a significantly decreased risk for myocardial infarction compared to the risk with conventional treatment, no statistical difference was demonstrated compared to the risk with the sulfonylureas or insulin. Metformin was associated with less weight gain and fewer hypoglycemia episodes than were the sulfonylureas and insulin.[3] The UKPDS strongly suggests that glucose control is a major factor in reducing microvascular complications. While glycemic control is important in controlling myocardial infarction, control of the other risk factors is obviously also needed.

Currently, there are a large number of drugs available to clinicians involved in the management of type 2 diabetes patients. These agents differ significantly in their mechanisms of action, efficacy, and potential for adverse events. This chapter will review overall treatment guidelines for patients with type 2 diabetes as well as the strengths and weaknesses of new and established oral therapies indicated for the management of these individuals.

■ Overall Treatment Guidelines

Dietary modification and exercise are considered to be the primary treatment modalities for patients with type 2 diabetes. However, if a 3-month program of diet and exercise does not result in normal or nearly normal plasma glucose levels, treatment with an oral agent or insulin may be necessary. See the treatment algorithm for the management of patients with type 2 diabetes (Figure 6-1).[4]

■ Classes of Oral Agents Used for the Treatment of Patients with Type 2 Diabetes

The four major classes of oral agents used for the treatment of patients with type 2 diabetes are listed below. They differ in their mechanisms of action, therapeutic effects, and associated adverse events.

SECRETAGOGUES

Sulfonylureas

First-generation agents
- Acetohexamide (Dymelor)
- Chlorpropamide (Diabinese)
- Tolazamide (Tolinase)
- Tolbutamide (Orinase)

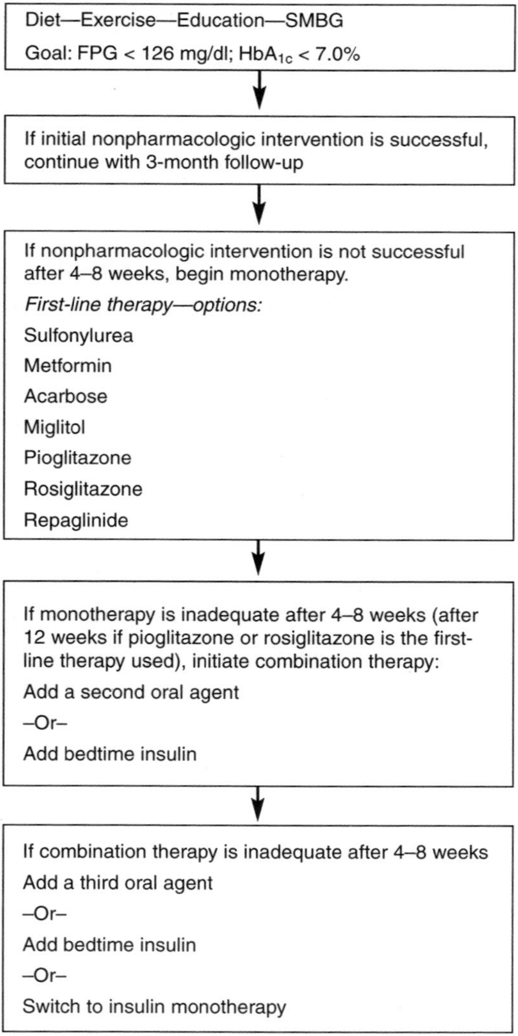

Diet—Exercise—Education—SMBG

Goal: FPG < 126 mg/dl; HbA$_{1c}$ < 7.0%

↓

If initial nonpharmacologic intervention is successful, continue with 3-month follow-up

↓

If nonpharmacologic intervention is not successful after 4–8 weeks, begin monotherapy.

First-line therapy—options:

Sulfonylurea

Metformin

Acarbose

Miglitol

Pioglitazone

Rosiglitazone

Repaglinide

↓

If monotherapy is inadequate after 4–8 weeks (after 12 weeks if pioglitazone or rosiglitazone is the first-line therapy used), initiate combination therapy:

Add a second oral agent

–Or–

Add bedtime insulin

↓

If combination therapy is inadequate after 4–8 weeks

Add a third oral agent

–Or–

Add bedtime insulin

–Or–

Switch to insulin monotherapy

Figure 6-1. Treatment Algorithm.[4] SMBG, self-monitored blood glucose.

Second-generation agents
- Glipizide (Glucotrol)
- Glipizide GITS (Glucotrol XL)
- Glimepiride (Amaryl)
- Glyburide (Micronase, Diaβeta, Glynase)

Meglitinides
- Repaglinide (Prandin)
- Nateglinide (Starlix)*

BIGUANIDES
- Metformin (Glucophage)

THIAZOLIDINEDIONES
- Rosiglitazone (Avandia)
- Pioglitazone (Actos)

ALPHA-GLUCOSIDASE INHIBITORS
- Acarbose (Precose)
- Miglitol (Glyset)

SECRETAGOGUES

Secretagogues are drugs that increase secretion of endogenous insulin. The two commonly used classes of these drugs are sulfonylureas and meglitinides. They stimulate insulin release by closing the K_{ATP} channel in the β-cell plasma membrane. Since the β-cell is the main site of action, secretagogues seem to be very effective in newly

---

* Starlix was approved by the FDA in December 2000.[42]

diagnosed type 2 diabetic patients. With progressive loss of β-cell function due to the natural history of type 2 diabetes, secretagogues may lose effectiveness over time, as, for example, in individuals with clinical diagnoses longer than 10 years. There is a wide variation in onset and duration of action among the drugs in this class.[5]

Sulfonylureas

The key characteristics of sulfonylureas are summarized in the list below.[6] More details are provided later in the chapter.

Key Characteristics of Sulfonylureas Used to Treat Type 2 Patients

Mechanism of Antihyperglycemic Action
- Increased insulin production and secretion of insulin by pancreatic β-cells
- Reduction of hepatic insulin resistance
- Reduction of peripheral insulin resistance

Therapeutic Efficacy
- May lower HbA_{1c} by 1–2%
- 70% of patients will respond initially
- After 5 years, 40% of responders maintain adequate glycemic control

Safety
- Most common clinically significant side effect is mild hypoglycemia

Hypoglycemia may occur with increased exercise, delayed meals, or both. These episodes are generally mild and easily treated with food.[6] As observed in the UKPDS, sulfonylureas have a tendency to promote weight gain. It appears that a major difference between first- and second-generation agents may be in the basal or fasting insulin levels achieved. Specifically, there appear to be differences in insulin levels between glyburide and glipizide because glyburide is more prone to continuous release of insulin, even during states of fasting.[7] Whether the hyperinsulinemia contributes to the weight gain is of great interest. There is evidence, however, that agents that do not seem to raise fasting insulin levels, such as glipizide GITS (Glucotrol XL), have a more favorable effect on weight gain.[8,9] In a head-to-head study with metformin, glipizide GITS and metformin were comparable as monotherapy on glucose control and body weight. Further, combination therapy was more effective than any agent alone.[10]

Meglitinides

The key characteristics of the meglitinides are summarized below.[11] More details are provided later in this chapter.

Key Characteristics of Meglitinides Used to Treat Type 2 Patients

Mechanism of Hypoglycemic Action
- Stimulates the release of insulin from the pancreas

Therapeutic Efficacy
- May reduce HbA_{1c} by 1%
- Compared to other secretagogues, may be associated with less hypoglycemia

Safety
- Most common clinical complaint is hypoglycemia

Common adverse events reported in placebo trials (12 to 24 weeks) and in comparative trials versus glyburide and glipizide (1 year) were hypoglycemia, hyperglycemia, upper respiratory tract infection, sinusitis, headache, and muscle pain.[11]

BIGUANIDES

The key characteristics of biguanides are summarized in the list below.[12–14] More details are provided later in the chapter.

Key Characteristics of Biguanides Used to Treat Type 2 Patients

Mechanism of Antihyperglycemic Action[12,13]

- Decreased hepatic gluconeogenesis
- Reduction of peripheral insulin resistance

Therapeutic Efficacy[14,15]

- May reduce HbA_{1c} by 1–2%
- Not significantly more effective than sulfonylureas as monotherapy with respect to glycemic control

Safety

- Most common clinical complaints involve the gastrointestinal system
- May result in lactic acidosis in a very small percentage (< 0.1%) of patients

Most of the adverse events associated with the use of the currently available biguanides in patients with type 2 diabetes involve the gastrointestinal system and include nausea, vomiting, and cramping. Lactic acidosis occurs only rarely (< 0.1% of patients).[13]

THIAZOLIDINEDIONES

The key characteristics of thiazolidinediones are summarized in the list below.[16–18] Additional information about thiazolidinediones is provided later in the chapter.

Key Characteristics of Thiazolidinediones Used to Treat Type 2 Patients

Mechanism of Antihyperglycemic Action[17,18]

- Reduction of peripheral insulin resistance
- Decreased hepatic gluconeogenesis

Therapeutic Efficacy[17,18]

- May lower HbA_{1c} by 0.3–1.9% when used as monotherapy or in combination with a sulfonylurea or insulin

Safety[16]

- Most common adverse events include respiratory tract infections and headache; in addition, patients on these drugs experienced weight gain, anemia, and edema
- Hypoglycemia has been noted in a small number of patients
- Liver function should be monitored periodically

Pending availability of long-term data from large-scale clinical trials, periodic monitoring of alanine aminotransferase (ALT) levels is advised.[17,18]

ALPHA-GLUCOSIDASE INHIBITORS

The key characteristics of alpha-glucosidase inhibitors are summarized in the list below.[6,19,20] Additional information about alpha-glucosidase inhibitors is provided later in the chapter.

Key Characteristics of Alpha-Glucosidase Inhibitors Used to Treat Type 2 Patients

Mechanism of Antihyperglycemic Action[6,19,20]

- Decreased breakdown and absorption of carbohydrates in the intestines
- Major effect is a decrease in postprandial glucose—thus, a reduction in overall glucose levels

Therapeutic Efficacy[19–21]

- Generally lowers HbA_{1c} by 0.5–1%

Safety[6]

- Most common side effects are gastrointestinal symptoms including cramping, diarrhea, and flatulence

The most common clinically significant side effects of alpha-glucosidase inhibitor therapy involve the gastrointestinal system and may occur in up to 40% of patients. The adverse events observed most often are cramping, flatulence, and diarrhea; all of these events are generally mild and tend to ameliorate with continued therapy.[6]

■ Key Properties of Individual Agents

This section summarizes the key properties of currently available members of each of the classes of agents listed in the preceding section.

SECRETAGOGUES

Sulfonylureas

Compared with the other classes of oral agents, sulfonylureas contain a relatively large number of drug choices. There have been two distinct generations in the development of these drugs. The first consisted of acetohexamide, chlorpropamide, tolazamide, and tolbutamide.[22] These drugs have been supplanted by more potent and better-tolerated second-generation drugs that include glyburide, glipizide (available in both immediate-release and long-acting GITS formulations), and glimepiride. Table 6-1 summarizes the key features of each second-generation drug of this class. The individual descriptions for each of these drugs are not intended to be exhaustive. Rather, key points for each agent are highlighted.

Glipizide GITS
The controlled-release formulation of glipizide, glipizide GITS, offers a distinct advantage over immediate-release glipizide with respect to duration of action.

Pharmacokinetics
The glipizide GITS formulation releases glipizide at a controlled rate into the gastrointestinal lumen regardless of pH or gastroin-

testinal motility. This formulation allows glipizide GITS to be administered once per day.[16] Administration of glipizide GITS immediately before a high-fat breakfast significantly increased bioavailability as reflected by maximum concentration (C_{max}). Reduced gastrointestinal retention time (occurring, for example, with short bowel syndrome) may reduce absorption of glipizide from the glipizide GITS formulation.[16]

Efficacy

Clinical trial results indicate that treating patients with type 2 diabetes using once-daily doses of glipizide GITS ranging from 5 to 60 mg resulted in 1.5–1.82% decreases in HbA_{1c}. Fasting plasma glucose also decreased from 57 to 74 mg/dl.[23] Compared to immediate-release formulations, glipizide GITS therapy also significantly reduced postprandial plasma glucose (PPG), insulin, and C-peptide.[24] Moreover, glipizide GITS did not appear to elevate fasting insulin levels.[9] The positive effects of glipizide GITS therapy were maintained for up to 12 months in 81% of patients in long-term extension trials.[16]

Treatment with glipizide GITS did not result in either weight gain or adverse effects on serum lipids.[23] As outlined previously, in a head-to-head study with metformin, glipizide GITS had comparable efficacy as monotherapy, and no difference between agents was observed on body weight.[10]

Safety

Results from controlled clinical trials indicate that the adverse events most often associated with glipizide GITS therapy versus placebo are asthenia (10.1% versus 13.0%), headache (8.6% versus 8.7%), dizziness (6.8% versus 5.8%), nervousness (3.6% versus 2.9%), tremor (3.6% versus 0%), diarrhea (5.4% versus 0%), and flatulence (3.2% versus 1.4%).[16] Further, hypoglycemia (blood glucose levels < 60 mg/dl and/or symptoms believed to be associated with hypoglycemia) occurred in 3.4% of patients treated with glipizide GITS in clinical trials.[16]

			TABLE 6-1 Key Features of Secretagogues: Currently Available Second-Generation Sulfonylureas and Meglitinides[6,11,16,23,25–31]			

Agent	Dose	Dosing Interval	Pharmacokinetic Considerations and Dosing Adjustments
Glipizide (Glucotrol)	Starting dose = 5 mg Maximum recommended dose = 40 mg	Once daily or in divided doses (divided doses should be used for total daily dose > 15 mg)	The starting dose should be 2.5 mg in geriatric patients or in those with liver disease
Glipizide GITS (Glucotrol XL)	Starting dose = 5 mg Maximum recommended dose = 20 mg	Once daily	The pharmacokinetics and pharmacodynamics of glipizide GITS may be affected by renal or hepatic impairment Gastrointestinal disease may also affect the pharmacokinetic profile and efficacy of glipizide GITS No dosing adjustment is required in the elderly (2.5 mg available)
Glimepiride (Amaryl)	Starting dose = 1 or 2 mg Maximum recommended dose = 8 mg	Once daily	A starting dose of 1 mg should be used in patients with renal impairment No dosing adjustment is required in the elderly

Abbreviation: FPG, fasting plasma glucose.

HbA$_{1c}$ Reduction	Durability of Efficacy	Contraindications	Most Common Adverse Events
1–2%	Effects of glipizide on HbA$_{1c}$ were maintained for 15 months, but the effect of treatment on FPG decreased between 3 and 15 months of therapy	Hypersensitivity to the drug Diabetic ketoacidosis (should be treated with insulin)	Most common adverse event in placebo-controlled clinical trials: hypoglycemia; other common adverse events in placebo-controlled trials involved the gastrointestinal system and included nausea and diarrhea
1.5–1.82%	Positive effects of glipizide GITS therapy were maintained for up to 12 months in 81% of patients in a long-term extension of a controlled clinical study	Hypersensitivity to the drug Diabetic ketoacidosis (should be treated with insulin)	Most common adverse event in placebo-controlled clinical trials: hypoglycemia; other common adverse events in placebo-controlled trials: asthenia, headache, dizziness, nervousness, tremor, diarrhea, and flatulence
1–1.5%	No meaningful reduction as an effect of glimepiride on either FPG or HbA$_{1c}$ was observed in patients treated for 2.5 years	Hypersensitivity to the drug Diabetic ketoacidosis (should be treated with insulin)	Most common adverse event in placebo-controlled clinical trials: hypoglycemia; other common adverse events in placebo-controlled trials: dizziness, asthenia, headache, and nausea

(Table continues)

TABLE 6-1 *(Continued)*
Key Features of Secretagogues:
Currently Available Second-Generation Sulfonylureas and Meglitinides[6,11,16,23,25-31]

Agent	Dose	Dosing Interval	Pharmacokinetic Considerations and Dosing Adjustments
Glyburide (Micronase, Diaβeta, Glynase)	Starting dose = 2.5–5 mg Maximum recommended dose = 20 mg	Once daily or in divided doses (divided doses may be most appropriate in patients taking >10 mg/day)	In elderly patients and patients with impaired renal or hepatic function, dosing should be conservative to avoid hypoglycemia
Repaglinide (Prandin)	Starting dose if not previously treated or HbA$_{1c}$ < 8% = 0.5 mg Previously treated or HbA$_{1c}$ ≤ 8% = 1 or 2 mg Maximum daily dose = 16 mg	Effective if given at the start of a meal, 15 minutes or 30 minutes before the meal	Allow one week to assess response to dose adjustment Use caution in patients with impaired liver function, with longer dose adjustment intervals

Glimepiride

Pharmacokinetics

Glimepiride is a once-daily drug with an elimination half-life of about 9 hours after multiple doses in patients with type 2 diabetes. Patient age has no significant effect on the pharmacokinetics of glimepiride, but the elimination half-lives of its metabolites are increased in patients with renal insufficiency. As a result, it is recommended that patients with renal impairment be started on 1 mg/day

HbA$_{1c}$ Reduction	Durability of Efficacy	Contraindications	Most Common Adverse Events
1–2%	Effects of glyburide on HbA$_{1c}$ were maintained for 15 months, but the effect of treatment on FPG decreased between 3 and 15 months of therapy	Hypersensitivity to the drug Diabetic ketoacidosis (should be treated with insulin)	Most common adverse event in placebo-controlled clinical trials: hypoglycemia; other common adverse events in placebo-controlled trials: nausea, vomiting, heartburn, and diarrhea
1–2%	Effects of repaglinide on HbA$_{1c}$ maintained for 24 weeks	Type 1 diabetes: diabetic ketosis Known hypersensitivity to the drug	Most common adverse events in placebo-controlled trials: hypoglycemia, upper respiratory tract infections, sinusitis, muscle pain, headache, weight gain

glimepiride. Administration with food slightly increases both the maximum plasma concentration (C_{max}) and AUC for glimepiride.[16]

Efficacy

The results of a large-scale clinical trial using a 14-week treatment regimen with 8 or 16 mg/day of glimepiride showed reductions in HbA$_{1c}$ ranging from 0.1–0.8%, whereas placebo-treated patients in this trial experienced a 2.0% increase in this parameter.[32] Treatment with glimepiride also resulted in significant reductions in FPG, PPG, fasting and postprandial insulin, and fasting C-peptide. The effect of glimepiride on either FPG or HbA$_{1c}$ was maintained in patients treated for 2.5 years.[16]

Safety
Adverse events observed most often in glimepiride-treated patients versus placebo include dizziness (1.7% versus 0.3%), asthenia (1.6% versus 1.0%), headache (1.5% versus 1.4%), and nausea (1.1% versus 0.0%).[16] Hypoglycemia (blood glucose < 60 mg/dl) occurred in 0.9–1.7% of patients treated with glimepiride in controlled clinical trials.[16]

Glyburide
Pharmacokinetics
Twenty-four hour serum levels are the same with a once-daily dosing of 6 mg or twice-daily dosing with 3 mg of glyburide. There is also no significant difference between the two treatments with respect to effects on FPG.[16] Co-ingestion of food does not alter either the rate of absorption or bioavailability of glyburide.[33]

The elimination of glyburide is decreased in patients with renal insufficiency. It has been suggested that glyburide should not be administered to patients with a creatinine clearance < 30 ml/min.[33,34] There have been no definitive studies of the effects of hepatic dysfunction on the pharmacokinetic profile for glyburide.[33]

Efficacy
The results of one clinical trial indicated that glyburide may lower HbA$_{1c}$ by as much as 2.1%.[16] In a 15-month trial, glyburide treatment resulted in an approximately 0.5% reduction in HbA$_{1c}$; the effect of glyburide on HbA$_{1c}$ was maintained for the duration of the study, but the effect of treatment on FPG decreased between 3 and 15 months of therapy.[25] Clinical trial results have also indicated that the effects of glyburide on indices of glycemic control are similar to those achieved with metformin.[14]

Safety

The adverse events most commonly associated with glyburide are nausea, vomiting, heartburn, and diarrhea. The overall rate of gastrointestinal side effects associated with glyburide has been reported to range between 0.5% and 1.8%. Hypoglycemia occurred in 1.6–3.1% of over 8,000 patients who were treated with glyburide.[26]

Meglitinides

Repaglinide

Repaglinide is currently the only meglitinide approved for treatment of type 2 diabetes (Table 6-1). It is also known as a benzoic acid derivative.

Pharmacokinetics

Clinical studies have shown that repaglinide taken with each meal results in a dose-proportional lowering of glucose over the full dose range. Insulin levels increase after meals and drop to baseline before the next meal. There is a linear relationship between dose and plasma drug levels. The drug is rapidly eliminated from the blood with an approximate half-life of 1 hour, providing a rapid onset and elimination. It is most effective when given three times a day before meals. When given with food, the T_{max} does not change, but the AUC decreases by 12.4%. The drug is metabolized by oxidative biotransformation and conjugation with glucuronic acid. Less than 2% of the unchanged drug is excreted in the feces, and 0.1% is cleared in the urine. Most of the drug is metabolized in the liver and excreted in the feces.[11]

Efficacy

Clinical trials have shown the efficacy of repaglinide as monotherapy and in combination. In a placebo-controlled, double-blind study over 3 months, patients treated with repaglinide had a 61 mg/dl lower FPG and a 104 mg/dl lower PPG concentration, compared to placebo. Compared to baseline, the FPG decreased 31 mg/dl and the PPG decreased 47.6 mg/dl. Compared to placebo, the repaglinide group had a 1.7% lower HbA$_{1c}$ concentration.[11]

In combination drug studies, repaglinide was used with metformin in 83 patients who had been unsatisfactorily managed with exercise, diet, and metformin. With combination therapy, the HbA$_{1c}$ improved by 1% unit, and the FPG decreased by 35 mg/dl.[11]

Safety

In clinical trials, hypoglycemia occurred in 16% of repaglinide patients, 20% of glyburide patients, and 19% of glipizide patients. Repaglinide should be administered with food to reduce the risk of hypoglycemia. Common adverse events reported with the use of repaglinide in placebo trials (12–24 weeks) and in trials comparing repaglinide with glyburide and glipizide (1 year) were hyperglycemia, upper respiratory tract infection, sinusitis, headache, and muscle pain. Caution and longer intervals between dose adjustments should be used in patients with hepatic dysfunction. The repaglinide AUC is weakly correlated to creatinine clearance, and increases in dosage should be made with caution in patients with renal impairment.[11]

BIGUANIDES

Metformin

Metformin is the only biguanide approved for the treatment of patients with type 2 diabetes in the United States. Table 6-2 summarizes its key features.

Pharmacokinetics

The pharmacokinetic profile of metformin requires twice-daily dosing.[16] The elimination half-life for this drug has been reported to range from 2–6 hours.[35] Food decreases the extent of and slightly delays the absorption of metformin. The AUC for metformin is reduced by 25% when it is taken with a meal.[16] Renal insufficiency delays the clearance of metformin and prolongs its elimination half-life. The half-life for metformin is also extended in elderly patients; therefore, conservative dosing is recommended in the elderly.[16]

Efficacy

Large-scale clinical studies of metformin indicated that metformin reduced the FPG by 52 mg/dl and HbA_{1c} by 1.4%. The effects of metformin therapy were sustained over 29 weeks. Metformin was not significantly more effective than the sulfonylureas were in reducing either the FPG or HbA_{1c}. However, the combination of these two agents was superior to either drug alone.*,[14] Metformin therapy also significantly lowered low-density lipoprotein cholesterol and had no significant negative effects on other plasma lipid fractions.[14]

Safety

The most common adverse events observed in patients receiving metformin were gastrointestinal symptoms including diarrhea, nausea, vomiting, abdominal bloating, flatulence, and anorexia. Metformin-associated adverse events may occur in as many as 30% of patients. In controlled studies, approximately 4% of subjects taking metformin discontinued therapy due to gastrointestinal symptoms.[16] In addition, lactic acidosis may occur in a very small percentage (< 0.1%) of patients.[6,15]

THIAZOLIDINEDIONES

Table 6-3 summarizes the key features of these agents.

---

* Recently the FDA approved a single-tablet combination of metformin and glyburide (Glucovance). The efficacy of this medication is similar to the combination of glyburide and metformin given as separate tablets.[43]

		TABLE 6-2 Key Features of Currently Available Biguanides[6,14,16]	
Agent	Dose	Dosing Interval	Pharmacokinetic Considerations and Dosing Adjustments
Metformin (Glucophage)	Starting dose = 500–850 mg Maximum recommended dose = 2500 mg Delivered in divided doses	Twice daily	The elimination half-life of metformin is increased and its clearance via the kidney is reduced in patients with renal insufficiency Elderly patients may also exhibit reduced metformin elimination It is recommended that both initial dosing and dose titration be conservative in the elderly as well as in those with renal dysfunction; it is also recommended that elderly patients not be titrated to the highest recommended metformin dose There have been no studies of metformin in patients with hepatic impairment

Pioglitazone

Pharmacokinetics

After oral administration, pioglitazone is measurable in serum within 30 minutes, with peak concentrations within 2 hours. Food delays the time to peak concentration up to 3–4 hours, without altering its absorption. The mean serum half-life of pioglitazone and total pioglitazone ranges from 3 to 7 hours and 16 to 24 hours, respectively. Steady state serum concentrations of pioglitazone are reached in 7 days. The drug is extensively metabolized by oxidation and hydroxylation, and metabolites are pharmacologically active. Approximately 15–30% of pioglitazone is recovered in the urine,

HbA$_{1c}$ Reduction	Durability of Efficacy	Contraindications	Most Common Adverse Events
1–2%	Positive effects of metformin therapy were maintained for at least 29 weeks in a controlled clinical study	Renal disease or dysfunction (serum creatinine ≥ 1.5 mg/dl in males and ≥ 1.4 mg/dl in females) Presence of iodinated contrast materials (for radiologic tests) that may alter renal function Hypersensitivity to the drug Acute or chronic metabolic acidosis	Most common adverse events are gastrointestinal symptoms including diarrhea, nausea, vomiting, abdominal bloating, flatulence, and anorexia. Lactic acidosis may occur in a very small percentage (< 0.1%) of patients

with most of the drug excreted into the bile, either unchanged or as metabolites, and eliminated in the feces.[17]

Efficacy

The efficacy of pioglitazone monotherapy was established with three randomized, double-blind, controlled trials of 16–26 weeks. Glycemia was controlled with a reduction in HbA$_{1c}$ from baseline of 0.8–1.9% and a reduction in FPG of 37–64 mg/dl, in naive patients. In previously treated patients, a reduction in HbA$_{1c}$ from baseline of 0.0–0.6% and a reduction in FPG of 27–55 mg/dl was seen.[17]

| | | | Pharmacokinetic |
| | | Dosing | Considerations and |
Agent	Dose	Interval	Dosing Adjustments
Pioglitazone (Actos)	Initiate at 15 mg or 30 mg Maximum daily dose = 45 mg	Should be taken once a day without regard to meal times	In patients with moderate to severe renal impairment, $t_{1/2}$ is unchanged No adjustment is advised for patients with renal impairment With hepatic dysfunction a 45% decrease in drug peak concentration is seen, without a change in AUC mean values Pioglitazone should not be used in patients with evidence of active liver disease or ALT > 2.5 times upper limit of normal
Rosiglitazone (Avandia)	Starting dose = 4 mg Maximum daily dose 8 mg QD	Single dose once a day or in divided doses twice daily	$t_{1/2}$ is about 2 hours longer in patients with liver disease If patient exhibits active liver disease or ALT > 2.5 times upper limit of normal, do not treat with rosiglitazone No dosage adjustments are needed in patients with mild to severe renal impairment

TABLE 6-3
Key Features of Currently Available Thiazolidinediones[17,18]

* From baseline.

HbA$_{1c}$ Reductions*	Durability of Efficacy	Contraindications	Most Common Adverse Events
0.3–1.9%	Based on open-label extension study data, glucose-lowering effects persist for at least 1 year	Hypersensitivity to the drug	Upper respiratory tract infections, headache, sinusitis, myalgia, tooth disorder, aggravation of diabetes, pharyngitis
0.1–0.7% as monotherapy; an additional 0.8–0.9% in combination therapy compared to monotherapy baseline	Improvement in glucose control was established, with maintenance of effect for 52 weeks	Hypersensitivity to the drug	Upper respiratory tract infections, back pain, anemia, edema

Safety

Adverse events reported at a frequency of ≥ 5% during clinical trials included upper respiratory tract infections, headache, sinusitis, myalgia, tooth disorder, aggravation of diabetes, and pharyngitis. Hypoglycemia was reported in 2% of patients when pioglitazone was used in combination with a sulfonylurea, compared to 1% with placebo. An increase in edema (pioglitazone 15% versus placebo 7%) was seen when pioglitazone was combined with insulin. With hepatic dysfunction, a 45% decrease in drug peak concentration was seen; therefore, pioglitazone should not be used in patients with evidence of an active liver disease or ALT > 2.5 times the upper limit of normal.[17] It is recommended that ALT levels be obtained at 2-month intervals during the first year and periodically thereafter.

Rosiglitazone

Pharmacokinetics

Rosiglitazone is extensively metabolized, and no unchanged drug is excreted in the urine. Its metabolites have low activity and are not expected to contribute to its insulin-sensitizing. The drug is mainly metabolized by cytochrome P450 isoenzyme 2C8, with CYP2CP as a minor pathway. The absolute bioavailability of the drug is 99%, and peak plasma concentrations are seen within 1 hour of dosing. Food induces a 28% decrease in C_{max} and a delay in T_{max} of 1.75 hours; however, these effects are not expected to be clinically significant, and rosiglitazone can be administered with or without food.[18]

Efficacy

The efficacy of monotherapy with rosiglitazone was established with three placebo-controlled trials of 26–52 weeks and three placebo-controlled, dose-ranging studies of 8–12 weeks. A total of 2,315 patients were involved in the studies. The trials demonstrated that the drug effectively controls glycemia with a significant placebo-adjusted reduction in HbA$_{1c}$ of 0.8–1.5% and a reduction in FPG from baseline of 25–55 mg/dl.[18] The combination of rosiglitazone with metformin resulted in a 0.8% reduction (from baseline) in HbA$_{1c}$ and a 48 mg/dl reduction in FPG. Combined with the sulfonylureas, rosiglitazone resulted in a 0.9% reduction in HbA$_{1c}$ and a 38 mg/dl reduction in FPG.[18]

Safety

The most common adverse event reported with rosiglitazone was upper respiratory tract infections (9.9% versus 8.7% for placebo, 8.9% for metformin, and 7.3% for sulfonylureas). Back pain, injury, and headache were reported at rates > 5%. A small number of patients were found to have anemia and edema of mild to moderate severity. Hypoglycemia was reported in 0.6% of patients, compared to 5.9% treated with sulfonylureas. Pending further studies, periodic monitoring of ALT levels is advised.[18]

ALPHA-GLUCOSIDASE INHIBITORS

Table 6-4 summarizes the key features of these agents.

Acarbose

Acarbose was the first alpha-glucosidase inhibitor indicated for the treatment of patients with type 2 diabetes in the United States.

Pharmacokinetics

The pharmacokinetic profile for acarbose requires thrice-daily dosing. The elimination half-life of this drug is approximately 2 hours.[16] Renal insufficiency markedly reduces the clearance of acarbose. Patients with severe renal impairment may have AUCs six times those observed in subjects with normal kidney function. As a result, acarbose is not recommended for treatment of patients with a serum creatinine > 2.0 mg/dl.[16]

	**TABLE 6-4** **Key Features of Currently Available Alpha-Glucosidase Inhibitors**[16,21,36,37]
Agent	Dose	Dosing Interval	Pharmacokinetic Considerations and Dosing Adjustments
Acarbose (Precose)	Starting dose = 25 mg Maximum recommended dose = 100 mg	Thrice daily	The elimination half-life of acarbose is 2 hours; this short elimination half-life results in the requirement for thrice-daily administration Both elderly patients and those with renal impairment are likely to experience higher plasma concentrations of acarbose; the elevations in the elderly are not clinically important, but those in patients with severe renal impairment may reach six times the levels noted in healthy volunteers Treatment with acarbose is not recommended in patients with serum creatinine > 2.0 mg/dl
Miglitol (Glyset)	Starting dose = 25 mg TID Maximum recommended dose = 100 mg TID	Three times a day at the start of each meal (with the first bite)	Miglitol is eliminated unchanged, by renal excretion Accumulation of drug is expected with renal impairment, therefore use of the drug with renal dysfunction is not recommended Hepatic impairment has no effect on drug kinetics

HbA$_{1c}$ Reduction	Durability of Efficacy	Contraindications	Most Common Adverse Events
0.56–0.78%	Positive effects of acarbose therapy have been maintained for at least 4 months in controlled clinical trials	Hypersensitivity to the drug Presence of diabetic ketoacidosis or cirrhosis, inflammatory bowel disease, colonic ulceration, intestinal obstruction, chronic intestinal disease, disorders of digestion, or any disease exacerbated by the presence of gas in the intestine	Most common adverse events are gastrointestinal symptoms including diarrhea, abdominal pain, and flatulence
0.22–0.84%	Positive effects have been shown in controlled fixed-dose monotherapy studies of up to 1 year	Diabetic ketoacidosis Inflammatory bowel disease, colonic ulceration, partial intestinal obstruction or predisposition to intestinal obstruction Chronic intestinal diseases Hypersensitivity to this drug	Abdominal pain, diarrhea, flatulence, skin rash, low serum iron

Efficacy

Clinical trial results have demonstrated that monotherapy with acarbose reduces FPG by 9–20 mg/dl and HbA_{1c} by 0.56–0.78%. These same studies demonstrated that acarbose reduced PPG by 34–38 mg/dl.[36] The addition of acarbose to a sulfonylurea produced a 0.54% reduction in HbA_{1c} over that observed with monotherapy.[16]

Safety

The most common adverse events reported for patients receiving acarbose involve the gastrointestinal system. They include flatulence (8–14% versus 7% for placebo), abdominal pain (3–4% compared with 0% for placebo), and diarrhea (0–1% versus 0% for placebo). The overall rate of adverse events for acarbose is 32–63% versus 31% for placebo.[37]

Miglitol

Pharmacokinetics

Miglitol is eliminated unchanged by renal excretion. An accumulation of the drug is expected with renal impairment; therefore, the use of miglitol in patients with renal dysfunction is not recommended. Hepatic impairment has no effect on the kinetics of miglitol.

Efficacy

The efficacy of miglitol monotherapy was demonstrated in 5 controlled, fixed-dose studies, involving 735 patients. In all studies, significant reductions in PPG were noted. A reduction in mean baseline HbA_{1c} of 0.26–1.02% (adjusted for treatment effect) was seen in all 5 trials.[21] In combination therapy trials, miglitol was evaluated as adjuvant therapy in patients with maximal or near-maximal sulfonylurea treatment. A reduction in HbA_{1c} of 0.30–0.82% (adjusted for treatment effect) was seen in 3 large, double-blind, randomized trials with 471 patients.[21]

Safety

The most common adverse reactions to miglitol are gastrointestinal abdominal pain (11.7%), diarrhea (28.7%), and flatulence (41.5%). Skin rashes, which are usually transient, are seen in 4.3%. Low serum iron was seen at a higher rate than that for placebo (9.2% versus 4.2%); however, it was not persistent and was not associated with changes in hemoglobin.[21] An accumulation of the drug is expected with renal impairment because miglitol is eliminated unchanged through renal excretion. The use of miglitol in patients with renal dysfunction is therefore not recommended. Hepatic impairment has no effect on drug kinetics.[21]

■ Choice of Initial Therapy

The choice of initial therapy is influenced by numerous factors. Based on the above descriptions of agents, it is apparent that all classes of agents demonstrate the ability to effectively lower glycemic control, but they differ in their side-effect profiles, mechanisms of action, and costs. Thus, these factors will obviously affect the treatment decision. However, whether one class is more beneficial than another as initial monotherapy has been debated. One study that addressed this issue was the UKPDS.[38] This study, begun in the late 1970s, randomized new-onset, type 2 subjects to either diet alone, a sulfonylurea, metformin, or insulin. Unfortunately, two classes of agents, thiazolidinediones and alpha-glucosidase inhibitors, were not yet commercially available and were not represented. The results of the study suggested that all types of pharmacologic monotherapy worked better than diet alone on glycemic control.[2,3] Further, there appeared to be no difference in the degree of initial glycemic response to the different types of pharmacologic monotherapy, and there also appeared to be very similar failure rates for all drug groups used as monotherapy. The study strongly suggested that all agents are comparable as initial therapy for glycemic control. Thus, when the initial monotherapy fails, combination therapy with other classes could be the next step. Combination therapy, as outlined in Figure 6-1, has shown great clinical promise (see Chapter 4 for more information).

■ Summary

The results summarized and tabulated in the preceding sections indicate that there are a number of effective oral therapies for patients with type 2 diabetes. While diet and exercise remain the cornerstones of treatment for these patients,[39] most are likely to require drug therapy.[40] All of the agents described above are indicated as monotherapy for patients with type 2 diabetes and have been shown to be effective in clinical trials.[16] However, monotherapy will not likely control the patient's symptoms over a prolonged period. If monotherapy failure should occur, combinations of agents (e.g., metformin and a sulfonylurea, a sulfonylurea and a thiazolidinedione) may permit achievement of glycemic control in some patients. Others may require the combination of an oral agent with insulin. Physicians must closely monitor glycemic control in patients with type 2 diabetes and alter treatment regimens as necessary to avoid the long-term consequences of hyperglycemia.[41]

■ References

1. Diabetes Control and Complications Trial Research Group. The effect of intensive treatment of diabetes on the development and progression of long-term complications in insulin-dependent diabetes mellitus. *N Engl J Med.* 1993;329:977–986.

2. UK Prospective Diabetes Study (UKPDS) Group. Intensive blood-glucose control with sulphonylureas or insulin compared with conventional treatment and risk of complications in patients with type 2 diabetes (UKPDS 33). *Lancet.* 1998;352:837–853.

3. UK Prospective Diabetes Study (UKPDS) Group. Effect of intensive blood-glucose control with metformin on complications in overweight patients with type 2 diabetes (UKPDS 34). *Lancet.* 1998;352:854–865.

4. DeFronzo RA. Pharmacologic therapy for type 2 diabetes mellitus. *Ann Intern Med.* 1999;131:281–303.

5. Lebovitz HE. Insulin secretagogues: old and new. *Diabetes Rev.* 1999;7:139–153.

6. Hollander PA. New oral agents for type II diabetes: taking a more aggressive approach to therapy. *Diabetes.* 1995;98:110–126.

7. Burge MR, Schmitz-Fiorentino K, Fischette C, Qualls CR, Schade DS. A prospective trial of risk factors for sulfonylurea-induced hypoglycemia in type 2 diabetes mellitus. *JAMA.* 1998;279(2):137–143.

8. Blonde L, Guthrie R, Tive L, Fischette C. Glipizide GITS is effective and safe in a wide range of NIDDM patients: results of a double-blind, placebo-controlled efficacy and safety trial. *Diabetes.* 1996;45:S2. Abstract 1054.

9. Cefalu WT, Bell-Farrow A, Wang ZQ, et al. Effect of glipizide GITS on insulin sensitivity, glycemic indices, and abdominal fat composition in NIDDM. *Drug Dev Res.* 1998;44:1–7.

10. Cefalu WT, Bell-Farrow AD, Terry JG, Wang ZQ, King T. Abdominal fat distribution with combination glipizide GITS/metformin treatment in type 2 diabetics. In: American Diabetes Association 59th Annual Meeting and Scientific Sessions. June 18–22, 1999; San Diego, Calif. Abstract #0344.

11. Prandin (repaglinide tablets) [prescribing information]. Princeton, NJ: Novo Nordisk.

12. Dunn CJ, Peters DH. Metformin: a review of its pharmacological properties and therapeutic use in non-insulin-dependent diabetes mellitus. *Drugs.* 1995; 49:721–749.

13. Lee AJ. Metformin in noninsulin-dependent diabetes mellitus. *Pharmacotherapy.* 1996;16:327–351.

14. DeFronzo RA, Goodman AM, The Multicenter Metformin Study Group. Efficacy of metformin in patients with non-insulin-dependent diabetes. *N Engl J Med.* 1995;333:541–549.

15. Wildasin EM, Skaar DJ, Kirchain WR, Hulse M. Metformin, a promising oral antihyperglycemic for the treatment of noninsulin-dependent diabetes mellitus. *Pharmacotherapy.* 1997;17:62–73.

16. *Physicians' Desk Reference.* Montvale, NJ: Medical Economics, 2000.

17. Actos (pioglitazone hydrochloride tablets) [prescribing information]. Indianapolis, Ind: Eli Lilly and Company. Available at: http://www.actos.com/pi. htm. Accessed August 16, 2000.

18. Avandia (rosiglitazone maleate tablets) [prescribing information]. Philadelphia, Pa: SmithKline Beecham. Available at: http://www.sb.com/cgi-bin/prescribing_information/2000b.cgi?drug=av. Accessed August 16, 2000.

19. Campbell LK, White JR, Campbell RK. Acarbose: its role in the treatment of diabetes mellitus. *Ann Pharmacotherapy.* 1996;30:1255–1262.

20. Yee HS, Fong NT. A review of the safety and efficacy of acarbose in diabetes mellitus. *Pharmacother.* 1996;16:792–805.

21. Glyset (miglitol tablets) [prescribing information]. Kalamazoo, Mich: Pharmacia & Upjohn.

22. Lebovitz HE. The oral hypoglycemic agents. In: Porte D Jr, Sherwin RS, eds. *Ellenberg & Rifkin's Diabetes Mellitus.* 5th ed. New York, NY: McGraw-Hill; 1997: 761–788.

23. Simonson DC, Kourides IA, Feinglos M, et al. Efficacy, safety, and dose-response characteristics of glipizide gastrointestinal therapeutic system on glycemic control and insulin secretion in NIDDM: results of two multicenter, randomized, placebo-controlled clinical trials. *Diabetes Care.* 1997;20:597–606.

24. Berelowitz M, Fischette C, Cefalu W, et al. Comparative efficacy of a once-daily controlled-release formulation of glipizide and immediate-release glipizide in patients with NIDDM. *Diabetes Care.* 1994;17:1460–1464.

25. Birkeland KI, Mowinckel P, Furuseth K, et al. Long-term randomized placebo-controlled double-blind therapeutic comparison of glipizide and glyburide. *Diabetes Care.* 1994;17:45–49.

26. Kolterman OG. Glyburide in non-insulin-dependent diabetes: an update. *Clin Ther.* 1992;14:196–213.

27. Draeger E. Clinical profile of glimepiride. *Diabetes Res Clin Pract.* 1995;28: S139–S146.

28. Rosenstock J, Corrao PJ, Goldbert RB, Kilo C. Diabetes control in the elderly: a randomized, comparative study of glyburide versus glipizide in non-insulin-dependent diabetes mellitus. *Clin Ther.* 1993;15:1031–1040.

29. Carlson RF, Isley WL, Ogrinc FG, Klobucar TR. Efficacy and safety of reformulated, micronized glyburide tablets in patients with non-insulin-dependent diabetes mellitus: a multicenter, double-blind, randomized trial. *Clin Ther.* 1993; 15:788–796.

30. Feldman JM. Review of glyburide after one year on the market. *Am J Med.* 1985;79:102–108.

31. Juan D, Molitch ME, Johnson MK, et al. Unaltered drug metabolizing enzyme systems in type II diabetes mellitus before and during glyburide therapy. *J Clin Pharmacol.* 1990;30:943–947.

32. Rosenstock J, Schneider J, Samols E, et al. Glimepiride, a new once-daily sulfonylurea. *Diabetes Care*. 1996;19:1194–1199.

33. Pearson JG. Pharmacokinetics of glyburide. *Am J Med*. 1985;79:67–71.

34. Harrower ADB. Pharmacokinetics of oral antihyperglycaemic agents in patients with renal insufficiency. *Clin Pharmacokinet*. 1996;31:111–119.

35. Scheen AJ. Clinical pharmacokinetics of metformin. *Clin Pharmacokinet*. 1996; 30:359–371.

36. Coniff R, Krol A. Acarbose: a review of US clinical experience. *Clin Ther*. 1997;19:16–26.

37. Santeusanio F, Compagnucci P. A risk-benefit appraisal of acarbose in the management of non-insulin-dependent diabetes mellitus. *Drug Saf*. 1994;11:432–444.

38. United Kingdom Prospective Diabetes Study Group. United Kingdom Prospective Diabetes Study 24: a 6-year randomized, controlled trial comparing sulfonylurea, insulin, and metformin therapy in patients with newly diagnosed type 2 diabetes that could not be controlled with diet therapy. *Ann Intern Med*. 1998;128:165–175.

39. Tan GH, Nelson RL. Concise review for primary-care physicians: pharmacologic treatment options for non-insulin-dependent diabetes mellitus. *Mayo Clin Proc*. 1996;71:763–768.

40. Baron AD, Prince MJ. Pathogenesis and management of early non-insulin-dependent diabetes mellitus. CME monograph at: Indiana University School of Medicine; 1996.

41. Harris P. Oral hypoglycaemic agents: when, how and why. *Aust Fam Physician*. 1997;26:391–396.

42. Starlix® (nateglinide) tablets [labeling information]. Available at: http://www.fda.gov/cder/approval/index.htm. Accessed March 7, 2001.

43. Glucovance (glyburide and metformin HCl tablets) [prescribing information]. Princeton, NJ: Bristol-Meyers Squibb Company. Available at: http://www.glucovance.com/Glucovanc.pdf. Accessed February 23, 2001.

CHAPTER SEVEN

Insulin Injection Therapy

■ Insulin Types

A level of plasma insulin at concentrations appropriate to the degree of insulin sensitivity is required for regulation of carbohydrate metabolism. In addition to its well-known role in stimulating glucose uptake into tissues, insulin is needed for metabolism of fat and protein. Insulin use, among both patients with type 1 diabetes and type 2 diabetes, must be individualized and balanced with diet and exercise. Available in rapid-, short-, intermediate-, and long-acting forms, the different types of insulin may be injected separately or mixed in the same syringe (Table 7-1).[1] Insulin is obtained from beef or pork pancreas and is made chemically identical to human insulin with recombinant DNA techniques or chemical modification of pork insulin.[2] On clinical grounds, animal-derived insulin has been observed to be more allergenic and to induce immune resistance; therefore, recombinant insulin has rapidly become a preferred formulation.[3]

In 1996, the FDA approved insulin lispro (Humalog), the first new insulin in 14 years and the first insulin analog. It was produced by switching the order of two amino acids—lysine and proline—in human insulin. This change allows insulin lispro to be absorbed and act more quickly than regular insulin, which was the fastest-acting insulin prior to lispro's approval. Due to its quick action,

TABLE 7-1
Insulin Types

Insulin type	Onset (hours)	Peak (hours)	Effective Duration (hours)	Maximum Duration (hours)
Rapid acting				
Human lispro	≤ 5 minutes	1	2–4	2–4
Insulin aspart[4]	≤ 5 minutes	40–50 minutes	3–5	3–5
Short acting				
Human regular	0.5–1.0	2–3	3–6	4–6
Intermediate acting				
Human NPH	2–4	4–10	10–16	14–18
Human lente	3–4	4–12	12–18	16–20
Long acting				
Insulin glargine[5]	1	None	10–19	11–24*
Human ultralente[12]	4–6	8–20	18–20	24–28

Note: Human insulins have a more rapid onset and shorter duration of activity than pork insulins, whereas beef insulins have the slowest onset and longest duration of activity.

*End of observation period.

(Modified from Kelley,[1] with permission.)

insulin lispro has the potential to induce hypoglycemia earlier after a meal. Hence, patients should take lispro no more than 5 to 15 minutes before a meal to match the rate at which blood glucose rises postprandially. Using insulin lispro may require the patient to take more injections, make dietary changes, and monitor blood glucose more frequently. Unlike most other insulins, lispro can now be purchased only with a prescription.[6]

In 2000, the rapid-acting insulin analog insulin aspart (NovoLog) was approved by the FDA. This product has faster absorption, faster onset, and a shorter duration than regular insulin.[4]

Also in 2000, insulin glargine (Lantus) was approved for human use. Insulin glargine is a long-acting (up to 24 hours' duration) recombinant human insulin analog for once-daily subcutaneous administration in the treatment of type 1 diabetes or type 2 diabetes. After this insulin is injected into subcutaneous tissue, microprecipitates form providing a slow release of insulin over 24 hours with no pronounced peak effect. Owing to its unique delivery characteristics, insulin glargine must not be mixed with other insulins or solutions.[5]

When transferring patients from once-daily NPH or ultralente insulin to once-daily glargine, initial dosing does not need modification. However, with a transfer from twice-daily NPH to daily glargine, the initial dose should be decreased approximately 20% within the first week of therapy and adjusted as needed to avoid hypoglycemia.[5]

Insulin is commercially available in concentrations of 100 or 500 U/ml, designated U-100 and U-500; 1 U = ~36 µg of insulin. Only in rare cases of insulin resistance, when the patient requires extremely large doses, is U-500 recommended. Like lispro, U-500 requires a prescription. Patients must purchase the correct syringe (i.e., one that matches the insulin concentration). For infants, insulin is sometimes formulated individually (e.g., U-10), with diluents provided by the manufacturer. The correct dose must be administered with an ordinary insulin syringe.[2]

EFFECTS ON ONSET, DEGREE, AND DURATION OF INSULIN ACTIVITY[2]

- Insulin type and species
- Injection technique
- Insulin antibodies
- Site of injection
- Individual patient response

Remind patients that when purchasing insulin they should make sure that the type and species are correct; that the specific brand prescribed is dispensed; and that the insulin will be used before the expiration date.[2]

■ Insulin Regimens

Total daily insulin dose should initially be based on body weight, activity level, and food intake. Adjustments after initial dosing should be based on home fingerstick glucose checks. There has

Indications for Insulin Therapy in Type 2 Patients

Presence of ketonuria in unstressed state
Nonobesity with persistently elevated glucose levels
Uncontrolled weight loss and hyperglycemia
Dehydration secondary to glycosuria and unresponsive to diet, oral
  agents, or both
Diet or oral agent failure with symptomatic hyperglycemia
Hyperglycemia, even without symptoms, unresponsive to diet or oral agents
Severe hypertriglyceridemia unresponsive to oral agents and diet

(From Porte D and Sherwin R, eds. *Ellenberg & Rifkin's Diabetes Mellitus*, 5th ed., 1997, McGraw-Hill.[7] Reproduced with permission of the McGraw-Hill Companies.)

been great debate on the use of sliding-scale regimens, and many would argue that such a regimen might not be ideal in managing glycemia.[8] Recently, the concept of carbohydrate counting has received considerable attention.[9] This regimen is designed to provide specific insulin requirements for every gram of carbohydrate consumed and, as such, mimics normal pancreatic response. For implementation, the patient is required to learn how to assess carbohydrate content in foods, to provide amounts on glucose records, and record insulin given along with glucose level achieved. After a review of the records, the provider will be able to provide a ratio (i.e., 1 U:15 g carbohydrate consumed) for that subject. With such records, adjustments in the ratio for each meal or activity level can be made. The various insulin regimens are described in Table 7-2.[2]

■ Insulin Use

Patients should consult a diabetes educator to learn how, when, and where to inject themselves. By mixing rapid- or short- and intermediate- or long-acting insulins, patients are more likely to attain a more normal glycemia than if they used a single insulin. Advise your patients to follow these ADA mixing guidelines*:

- If diabetes is well controlled on a particular mixed-insulin regimen, maintain the procedure.
- Do not mix any other medication or diluent with any insulin product without physician approval.
- Premixed insulins may be used if the insulin ratio is appropriate to patients' needs.

(Text continues on page 114.)

---

* Adapted from American Diabetes Association,[2] with permission.

TABLE 7-2
Design of Insulin Regimens

Insulin Regimen	Patient Selection/ Indications for Use	Advantages	Disadvantages	Self-monitoring
Single morning insulin injection	Newly diagnosed	Simple, easy to understand and administer	Hypoglycemia, especially nocturnal hypoglycemia, can occur with large doses	Blood glucose monitoring 1–2× daily or at least in acute situations
	End-stage renal disease on dialysis	Preparations of a mixture of intermediate and short-acting insulin are available	Insulin availability is inadequate at certain times	
	Physical disabilities (impaired vision, coordination) Limited motivation for diabetes management		Least effective regimen and rarely suitable	
Twice daily injection of intermediate-acting insulin alone or in combination with regular insulin	When single injection leads to hypoglycemia or inadequate glycemic control Patients with fairly consistent schedules Patients with limited physical/intellectual motivational capabilities	Relatively simple, especially if premixed (e.g., 70/30)* preparations are used Good insulin availability over 24-hour period Can provide algorithm to adjust regular insulin	Requires consistent routine Can result in late afternoon and nocturnal hypoglycemia with prebreakfast hyperglycemia Ratio of premixed (e.g.,	Blood glucose monitoring 2–4× daily

Regimen	Indications	Advantages	Disadvantages	Monitoring
Multiple daily insulin injections (MDI)	Unacceptable glycemic control on BID insulin (excessive hypo-/hyperglycemia) Wide and erratic blood glucose excursions	based on premeal blood glucose level	70/30)* intermediate and short-acting insulin may contain too much short-acting insulin for PM dose	Blood glucose requires monitoring 3–4× daily
Intermediate and short-acting insulin before breakfast, short-acting insulin before supper, intermediate-acting insulin at bedtime	More flexibility needed More patient involvement in management desired Sufficient physical and intellectual motivational capabilities Improved or near-normal glycemic control desired	Helps eliminate nocturnal hypoglycemia Can improve glycemic control Some added lifestyle flexibility Insulin algorithms for regular insulin based on premeal blood glucose level can be used	Additional injections	
Regular insulin before each meal, intermediate-acting insulin at bedtime	As above	Lifestyle can be more flexible Good insulin availability with each meal Basal needs provided for without nocturnal hypoglycemia	Regular insulin must be taken 4–6 hours apart	Blood glucose monitoring 4× daily before each injection

(Table continues)

111

TABLE 7-2 (Continued)
Design of Insulin Regimens

Insulin Regimen	Patient Selection/ Indications for Use	Advantages	Disadvantages	Self-monitoring
Intermediate and short-acting insulin before breakfast, regular insulin before lunch and supper, intermediate-acting insulin before bedtime	As above, but patient is inconsistent or misses premeal regular injection at lunch	Provides 24-hour basal needs and does not rely on regular insulin at proper intervals	As above	Blood glucose monitoring 4× daily
Regular or fast-acting insulin before each meal with Ultralente insulin pre-breakfast and/ or pre-supper	As above	More flexibility Good insulin availability with each meal	Additional injections required Regular insulin should be taken 4–6 hours apart Ultralente may have unpredictable peaks of action	Blood glucose monitoring 4× daily before each injection

| Continuous subcutaneous insulin infusion (CSII): regular insulin via continuous basal rate and premeal bolus | As for MDI Sufficiently motivated, healthy, and capable to integrate the technical and problem-solving skills needed to safely employ the insulin pump | Maximum lifestyle flexibility Insulin delivery like that of nondiabetic individual Reduces unpredictable absorption of depot insulin Use of insulin algorithms | Mechanical device must be worn 24 hours a day Potential for hyperglycemia/ketosis related to pump malfunction or interruption of insulin delivery Potential for infusion site infection Increased cost | Blood glucose monitoring 4× daily before each bolus |

Note: There are now several ratios of premixed.

(Modified from Porte D and Sherwin R, eds. *Ellenberg & Rifkin's Diabetes Mellitus*, 5th ed., 1977 McGraw-Hill.[10] Reproduced with permission of the McGraw-Hill Companies.)

- Currently available NPH and short-acting insulin preparations may be used immediately or stored for future use.
- When rapid-acting insulin is mixed with either an intermediate- or long-acting insulin, the mixture should be injected within 15 minutes before a meal.
- Mixing short-acting and zinc-containing lente insulins is not recommended except for patients whose diabetes is already adequately controlled on such a mixture; the zinc can delay onset of action.
- Phosphate-buffered insulins (e.g., NPH) should not be mixed with lente insulins; zinc phosphate may precipitate, and the longer-acting insulin will convert, unpredictably, to a short-acting insulin.
- Because insulin formulations can change, consult with the manufacturer in cases in which their recommendations conflict with ADA guidelines.

■ Syringe Alternatives

INSULIN PEN[11]

- Convenient for patients who take at least three doses of insulin a day
- Cartridge holds 100–200 U of insulin
- Users turn a dial to select the desired dose of insulin and press a plunger to deliver the drug
- Provides great flexibility in lifestyle, meal schedules, and travel
- Low-dose insulin pens are available that deliver insulin in increments of $1/2$ U. Currently there are no available syringes calibrated to $1/2$ U.[3]

■ External Insulin Pump (Continuous Subcutaneous Insulin Infusion [CSII])

The external insulin pump is an alternative to multiple daily injections for achieving near-normal glucose levels; however, undetected interruptions in insulin delivery may result in ketotic episodes. Infections or inflammation at the needle site may complicate pump therapy but can be minimized with careful hygiene and frequent site changes. Other aspects of the external insulin pump include the following[11]:

- Can provide greater flexibility in lifestyle, meal schedules, and travel
- Attaches to the body through flexible plastic tubing and a needle inserted subcutaneously near the abdomen
- Size of a deck of cards; weighs 4–6 oz; can be worn on a belt or in a pocket
- Refillable cartridge holds enough insulin for about 2 days
- Patient needs to change needle and tubing every 2 days
- User sets the pump to deliver a basal level of insulin continuously throughout the day; most pumps can be set at several different basal rates. At meal times, and when hyperglycemic, users can inject an insulin bolus.

Note: It is essential to monitor blood glucose frequently to determine whether the correct insulin dosage is being delivered.

■ Implantable Insulin Pump

Please refer to Chapter 9 for discussion of the implantable insulin pump.

■ References

1. Kelley DB, ed-in-chief. *American Diabetes Association Complete Guide to Diabetes.* Alexandria, Va: American Diabetes Association; 1996:96.
2. American Diabetes Association. Clinical Practice Recommendations 1998. Insulin administration. *Diabetes Care.* 1998;21(suppl 1)S72–S75.
3. American Diabetes Association. Clinical Practice Recommendations 2000. Insulin administration. *Diabetes Care.* 2000;23(suppl 1):S86–S89.
4. NovoLog™ (insulin aspart) labeling information. Available at http://FDA.gov/CDER/FOI/label/2000/20986lbl.pdf. Accessed August 14, 2000.
5. Lantus® (insulin glargine) prescribing information. Available at http://www.aventispharma-us.com/pis/lantus_txt.html. Accessed August 14, 2000.
6. McCarren M. A new faster insulin? It's here! *Diabetes Forecast.* 1996:49(8). Available at http://www.diabetes.org/diabetesforecast/96aug/wait.htm. Accessed October 30, 2000.
7. Nathan DM: Insulin treatment of noninsulin-dependent diabetes mellitus. In Porte D Jr., Sherwin RS, eds. *Ellenberg & Rifkin's Diabetes Mellitus.* 5th ed. New York, NY: McGraw-Hill; 1997:733–743.
8. Queale WS, Seidler AJ, Brancati FL. Glycemic control and sliding scale insulin use in medical inpatients with diabetes mellitus. *Arch Intern Med.* 1997; 157:545–552.
9. Gillespie SJ, Kularni KD, Daly AE. Using carbohydrate counting in diabetes clinical practice. *J Am Diet Assoc.* 1998;98:897–905.
10. Strowig S, Raskin P. Intensive management of insulin-dependent diabetes mellitus. In: Porte D Jr., Sherwin RS, eds. *Ellenberg & Rifkin's Diabetes Mellitus.* 5th ed. New York, NY: McGraw-Hill; 997:709–733.
11. National Institute of Diabetes and Digestive and Kidney Diseases (NIDDK). Devices for Taking Insulin. Available at http://www.niddk.nih.gov/health/diabetes/summary/altins/altins.htm. Accessed October 30, 2000.
12. *Pharmacist's Drug Handbook.* Springhouse, Penn.: Springhouse; and Bethesda, Md.: American Society of Health-System Pharmacists; 2001:608.

CHAPTER EIGHT

Standards of Care
for Patients With Diabetes

Over time many patients with diabetes will experience complications such as retinopathy, cardiovascular disease, nephropathy, and neuropathy, among others (see Chapter 3). However, with vigilance and rigorous treatment, progression of complications can be delayed, and morbidity minimized, allowing a good quality of life.

■ Retinopathy

SYMPTOMS

Retinopathy generally progresses from mild nonproliferative abnormalities with increased vascular permeability to moderate and severe nonproliferative diabetic retinopathy (NPDR) with vascular closure and then on to proliferative diabetic retinopathy (PDR) with new blood vessel growth on the retina and posterior surface of the vitreous. These changes can be accelerated by puberty, cataract surgery, or pregnancy.[1]

In the early stages, there are often no symptoms and no pain. Vision may not change until the disease has become severe. Macular edema or capillary nonperfusion can occur and impair central vision. New blood vessels of proliferative retinopathy and contraction of their accompanying fibrous tissue can distort the retina. This may lead to retinal detachment with severe and often irreversible vision loss. Further, the new blood vessels may bleed, which adds the complication of preretinal or vitreous hemorrhage.

DIAGNOSIS[1]

The ADA recommends yearly dilated ophthalmoscopic examination performed by an ophthalmologist or optometrist. Type 1 patients should be screened annually for retinopathy within 3 to 5 years after onset of diabetes. Type 2 patients should have an initial examination for retinopathy shortly after the diagnosis of diabetes has been established. Women with diabetes who become pregnant should have a comprehensive eye examination in the first trimester and be closely watched throughout their pregnancy. Women who develop gestational diabetes are not at increased risk for retinopathy and do not need the comprehensive eye examination and follow-up care.

TREATMENT

Laser photocoagulation therapy has established efficacy in preventing loss of vision in most patients with severe NPDR. Panretinal photocoagulation laser surgery is recommended for eyes approaching high-risk characteristics, such as disc neovascularization or vitreous hemorrhage with retinal neovascularization. Focal photocoagulation laser surgery has been established to be of benefit in eyes with macular edema, particularly when it is clinically significant.[1]

A qualified ophthalmologist can perform the procedure on an outpatient basis, usually over several visits. Although the therapy may reduce peripheral and night vision, its efficacy in preserving visual acuity probably outweighs the risks.

In advanced cases of retinopathy that may be associated with retinal hemorrhage, vitrectomy may be necessary. In many cases, this procedure can improve or stabilize vision.

Aspirin has not been found to prevent development of high-risk PDR or to reduce the risk of visual loss.[1]

■ Macrovascular Disease

Although diabetes itself is associated with an increased risk of coronary heart disease (CHD), commonly measured clinical factors, such as high-density lipoprotein (HDL) cholesterol, low-density lipoprotein (LDL) cholesterol, total cholesterol, triglycerides, and blood pressure, are highly predictive of macrovascular disorders

TABLE 8-1 Lipid Levels for Adults			
Risk for Adults with Diabetes	HDL Cholesterol (mg/dl)	LDL Cholesterol (mg/dl)	Triglycerides (mg/dl)
Low	> 45	< 100	< 200*
Borderline	35–45	100–129	200–399
High	< 35	≥ 130	≥ 400

*Because patients with evidence of macrovascular disease are at greatest risk for cardiovascular morbidity and mortality, they should strive to achieve an LDL cholesterol of ≤ 100 mg/dl and a triglyceride level of ≤ 200 mg/dl. This ADA recommendation is based on the results of intervention trials in patients without diabetes. It has been suggested that individuals with a cardiovascular history should have a target goal for LDL of < 100 mg/dl to reduce the chance of a second event (i.e., secondary prevention).

(Adapted from American Diabetes Association,[2] with permission.)

and should be used.[2–4] Table 8-1 lists the ADA-recommended levels for HDL and LDL cholesterol and triglycerides.

Several large studies have demonstrated that cholesterol-lowering therapy can significantly reduce coronary events. The Scandinavian Simvastatin Survival Study (4S) demonstrated that the use of simvastatin, a hydroxymethylglutaryl coenzyme A (HMG CoA) reductase inhibitor, resulted in a 35% mean reduction of LDL, reducing coronary mortality rates by 42% and total mortality rates by 30%.[5] In the Cholesterol and Recurrent Events (CARE) Study, pravastatin was shown to reduce fatal and nonfatal coronary events in patients with CHD,[6] and the West of Scotland Coronary Prevention (WOSCOP) Study Group presented similar results in persons without CHD.[7] In the Air Force/Texas Coronary Atherosclerosis Prevention Study (AFCAPS/TexCAPS), findings showed that lovastatin reduces the risk of first acute coronary events in individuals with average LDL cholesterol and triglyceride levels and below-average HDL cholesterol levels.[8]

Although the benefits of lipid-lowering treatment in reducing coronary mortality has been established in individuals who do not have diabetes, little data have been presented regarding the benefits in the at-risk group of patients with diabetes. Subgroup analysis of the 4S data demonstrated that treating individuals with diabetes with simvastatin reduced coronary events in hyperlipidemic patients by 55%. Based on the higher absolute risk of recurrent CHD events in patients with diabetes, the absolute clinical benefits of cholesterol lowering may be greater than in those without diabetes.[9] Subgroup analysis of the CARE trial showed that pravastatin is effective in reducing risk of CHD in persons with diabetes with normal cholesterol levels and in those with impaired fasting glucose levels. Pravastatin treatment resulted in a 25% risk reduction in coronary events in patients with diabetes and a 23% reduction in those without diabetes.[10]

LIPID DISORDERS

Like most patients with elevated cholesterol, patients with diabetes should attempt initially to curb this risk factor for macrovascular disease with diet and exercise—the same measures that can help improve glycemic control.[2]

After age 2 years, pediatric patients with diabetes should be tested for lipid disorders soon after diagnosis, and if any values are abnormal, annual testing should be performed.

Adult patients with diabetes should be tested for lipid disorders annually with a fasting serum cholesterol, triglyceride, HDL cholesterol, and calculated LDL cholesterol. When triglycerides are greater than 400 mg/dl, a calculated LDL level is not valid. In that case, every attempt should be made to improve glycemia, as improved glycemia (especially with use of insulin regimens) may markedly reduce triglycerides. If triglycerides remain elevated, a direct assessment of LDL can be made by the clinical laboratory.[11] If all values fall within lower-risk levels, the lipid profile may be obtained every 2 years.[2]

If the cholesterol and LDL cholesterol values are elevated, a serum thyroid stimulating hormone (TSH) should be measured to rule out hypothyroidism, a disorder not uncommon among diabetic patients. Co-existing disorders or conditions (such as smoking, hypertension, family history of premature CHD, and decreased HDL levels) that greatly increase the risk of cardiovascular disease in patients with diabetes should be factored into the consideration of target lipid levels. In adults with diabetes mellitus, ideal levels are LDL cholesterol < 100 mg/dl, HDL cholesterol > 45 mg/dl, and triglycerides < 200 mg/dl.[2] Patients with diabetes who have clinical CHD and an LDL cholesterol level > 100 mg/dl, despite medical nutrition therapy, exercise, and glucose control, should be treated with pharmacologic agents. Patients with diabetes who do not have CHD should be started on behavioral interventions, with the addition of drug therapy if LDL cholesterol remains ≥ 130 mg/dl and a goal of ≤ 100 mg/dl has been set.[2] Lowering LDL cholesterol is the first priority of drug therapy, on the basis of clinical data showing efficacy of statins in decreasing the risk of CHD in patients with diabetes. Table 8-2 lists available pharmacologic interventions.

Patients with diabetes who have triglyceride levels ≥ 1,000 mg/dl are at risk for pancreatitis. Severe dietary fat restrictions to < 10% of calories is needed in this group, along with pharmacotherapy. Improved glycemic control may also be effective in reducing triglyceride levels. The addition of a fibric acid may be considered after reaching optimal glycemic control.[2]

The ADA cautions physicians choosing a lipid-lowering agent for patients with diabetes to take into account several considerations, as discussed below.[12]

TABLE 8-2
Pharmacologic Management of Dyslipidemia in Adults

	Effect on Lipoprotein		
	LDL	HDL	Triglycerides
First-line agents			
LDL-lowering			
HMG-CoA reductase inhibitor	↓↓	↔↑	↔↓
Triglyceride-lowering			
Fibric acid derivative	↓↔↑	↑	↓↓
Second-line agents			
LDL-lowering			
Bile acid resins	↓	↔	↑
LDL- and triglyceride-lowering			
Nicotinic acid	↓	↑↑	↓↓

Symbols: ↓ decrease, ↑ increase, ↔ no change.

(Adapted from American Diabetes Association,[2] with permission.)

HMG-CoA Reductase Inhibitors

Clinical trials have shown convincing effectiveness of HMG-CoA reductase inhibitors, or statins, in decreasing CHD in individuals with diabetes.[2] The data from the CARE and 4S trials showed that absolute risk reduction with statin treatment was greater in those with diabetes than in those without it. Consequently, statins have been adopted as first-line therapy in controlling diabetic dyslipidemia.[13]

These drugs inhibit HMG-CoA reductase, which catalyzes the rate-limiting step in biosynthesis of cholesterol. They are superior to other lipid-lowering drugs in decreasing LDL and are moderately effective in increasing HDL. No modification of size and density of LDL is seen with these drugs.[13] In primary hypertriglyceridemia with elevated total cholesterol or LDL, a fibric acid derivative should be considered first.[14]

The choice of statin should be based on LDL reduction goals, initial LDL level, and clinical judgment. Laboratory findings should be used as the basis for dosage adjustment, at 4- to 6-week intervals.[2] The reduction in triglyceride level is directly proportional to baseline triglyceride level and the LDL-lowering potency of the drug used. In general, with each doubling of the dose from the starting dose of the drug, LDL will be reduced an additional 7%.[13]

Combining a statin with a bile acid–binding resin, which have different mechanisms of action to stimulate LDL receptor clearance of LDL, is highly effective for LDL lowering. Triple therapy with statin, resin, and niacin may occasionally be required to achieve lipid control. The efficacy of combinations of statin and fibrate or statin and niacin has not been addressed.[13]

Statins are generally well tolerated. The major adverse effects reported are liver and muscle toxicity, which presents as myopathy. Baseline and periodic monitoring of liver transaminases is recommended. Combining statins with drugs that are known CYP3A4 inhibitors or substrates increases the risk of myopathy. Additionally, fibrates and niacin increase the risk of statin-induced myopathy via a mechanism that does not increase plasma statin concentrations. Unfortunately, in many cases of diabetic dyslipidemia, triglycerides remain elevated despite statin therapy. In these cases, combination with fibrates may be considered, but the patient needs to be monitored carefully. If combination therapy is used, it is best to use lower doses of statins, if possible, as low doses of statins have been found to be safe in combination with niacin and fibrates.[13]

Bile Acid–Binding Resins

Agents such as colestipol and cholestyramine have been a long-standing choice and can elevate very-low-density lipoprotein (VLDL) and triglyceride levels. Such agents do not appear to adversely affect glucose levels.

Note: These drugs should be administered cautiously in the elderly or in diabetic patients with gastrointestinal autonomic neuropathy as they may produce constipation or even fecal impaction. They may also worsen hypertriglyceridemia.[14]

Fibric Acid Derivatives

Gemfibrozil has proven effective in lowering triglyceride levels in patients with diabetes. Overall, these agents generally do not have a marked LDL-lowering effect and therefore are usually not considered primary therapy for LDL elevation in type 2 diabetes. In addition, there appears to be minimal effect on glycemic control. Gemfibrozil should not be initiated alone in patients with both elevated triglyceride and elevated LDL cholesterol levels. Fenofibrate may be more effective in lowering LDL and treating mixed lipidemia.[2]

Nicotinic Acid

Niacin derivatives have favorable effects on lowering triglyceride levels and increasing HDL levels. Yet these agents can worsen glycemic control in patients with diabetes and their side effects generally limit their use to those patients who can tolerate them. Nicotinic acid may also adversely affect insulin sensitivity.[14] As it is relatively contraindicated in patients with diabetes, it should be restricted to < 2 g/day. Use of the short-acting nicotinic acid preparation is preferred.[2]

Estrogen

The risk of heart disease in premenopausal women is considerably less than in men. In the postmenopausal period, a woman's risk of heart disease increases significantly. Numerous population-based observational studies have confirmed estrogen's cardioprotective effects. However, in the Heart and Estrogen/Progestin Replacement Study (HERS), a recent prospective, secondary prevention trial done with 2,763 postmenopausal women with established CHD, a favorable effect of oral hormone replacement therapy (HRT) was not seen. Primary HERS outcomes were occurrence of nonfatal myocardial infarction or CHD death, and secondary cardiovascular outcomes were coronary revascularization, unstable angina, congestive heart failure (CHF), resuscitated cardiac arrest, stroke, transient ischemic attack, and peripheral arterial disease (PAD). A trend in increased risk of cardiovascular disease was seen in hormone-treated patients the first year. The results suggest that in some patients, the acute prothrombotic effects of oral estrogen may outweigh long-term antiatherosclerotic effects.[15]

The results of HERS were further substantiated by the Estrogen Replacement and Atherosclerosis (ERA) Trial, a double-blind, placebo-controlled study involving 309 women and examining the effects of hormone replacement therapy on coronary atherosclerosis progression. This study also found that estrogen did not affect the progression of atherosclerosis in women who already had the disease.[16] As indicated by these studies, use of HRT requires a careful examination of potential risks and benefits of therapy.

HYPERTENSION

The ADA recommends that the primary goal for adults is to attain a blood pressure of < 130/85 mm Hg. The risk of end-organ failure seems to be lowest when systolic blood pressure is < 120 mm Hg and the diastolic is < 80 mm Hg. In patients with systolic readings ≥ 180 mm Hg, an initial goal is < 160 mm Hg. If systolic blood pressure is 160 to 179, a reduction of 20 mm Hg is an appropriate goal, with the ideal being 140 mm Hg.[17]

Antihypertensive Agents

Physicians should urge patients with mild to moderate hypertension to try lifestyle modifications (weight reduction, exercise, smoking cessation, as well as improved glycemic control) for 3 months. If at the end of that period they cannot successfully control blood pressure, drug treatment should be added.

Few clinical data have been presented on the efficacy of the various classes of antihypertensive agents in diabetic patients. The UKPDS group studied the efficacy of a beta-blocker (atenolol) versus an angiotensin-converting enzyme (ACE) inhibitor (captopril) in reducing risk of complications of type 2 diabetes. The randomized controlled study, done with 1,148 individuals with hypertension and type 2 diabetes, showed no significant advantage of one drug over the other. Both drugs were equally effective in reducing blood pressure and reducing the risk of fatal and nonfatal diabetes complications, death related to diabetes, macrovascular end points (myocardial infarction, stroke, heart failure, peripheral vascular disease [PVD]), retinopathy, and renal failure.[18]

Choice of treatment must rely on data derived from current understanding of the pathophysiology of hypertension in diabetes and the known pharmacologic actions and side effects of the various agents. An ADA panel reached no consensus that any single class of antihypertensive drug is preferred as initial therapy for hypertension in diabetes in the absence of nephropathy. Each class of drugs has potential advantages and disadvantages.[19]

Thiazide Diuretics

Thiazide diuretics are effective in reducing the expanded plasma volume often associated with hypertension in patients with diabetes. If response is inadequate at the recommended dosage (12.5 to 25 mg hydrochlorothiazide or chlorthalidone daily), substitute or add another class of antihypertensive agents. These agents appear to act synergistically with other classes of antihypertensive agents to improve blood pressure levels. At higher doses, these agents can have adverse effects on both glucose and lipid levels.

Beta-Blockers

It was initially shown that beta-blockers can adversely affect glycemic control and lipid levels. However, use of selective beta$_1$-blockers appears to have minimal effects. Beta-blockers may also interfere with awareness of and recovery from hypoglycemia. Peripheral blood flow is reduced; claudication and vasospasm can worsen. However, these agents have been shown to offer cardio-protection following acute myocardial infarction.

Angiotensin-Converting Enzyme Inhibitors

ACE inhibitors have demonstrated favorable effects on reducing microalbuminuria and proteinuria, as well as cardiovascular risk factors. The Heart Outcomes Prevention Evaluation (HOPE) Study examined the effects of the ACE inhibitor ramipril on cardiovascular risk in 3,577 people with diabetes who had had a previous cardiovascular event or at least one cardiovascular risk factor in addition to their diabetes. The results showed that the ACE inhibitor had a beneficial effect on cardiovascular events and nephropathy in these patients.[20] As such, studies have suggested a delayed onset or retardation of diabetic nephropathy. There appears to be no adverse effect on glucose or insulin levels, and there has been evidence in some studies of improved insulin sensitivity. In the first weeks of therapy, serum potassium and creatinine need to be closely monitored.

Note: Rapid decline in kidney function can occur in patients with renal artery stenosis. ACE inhibitors are contraindicated in pregnant women and should be used with caution in women of childbearing age.

Calcium Antagonists

Calcium antagonists are widely used to treat hypertension and cardiovascular disease in both patients with and without diabetes. They do not adversely affect lipid levels or glycemic control. However, the long-term renal protective effects are not known. Possible side effects are constipation and peripheral edema.

Alpha₁-Receptor Blockers

Alpha$_1$-receptor blockers do not appear to have adverse effects on lipid or glucose levels, and some studies have suggested a beneficial effect on glycemic control. A possible side effect is orthostatic hypotension, particularly in diabetic patients with autonomic dysfunction.

■ Nephropathy

SYMPTOMS[21,22]

Symptoms of nephropathy usually occur only in late stages of the disease, when kidney function has fallen to less than 25% of normal. One of the first detectable signs is microalbuminuria (> 30 mg/day or 20 µg/min). Without intervention, this level can progress to clinical albuminuria ($\geq$ 300 mg/24 h or ~200 µg/min) over 10 to 15 years, with hypertension developing along the way. Without intervention, overt nephropathy and end-stage renal disease (ESRD) may develop.

DIAGNOSIS[22]

Screen patients annually for microalbuminuria. Adult patients should have routine urinalysis. In type 1 patients, screening should begin at puberty or 5 years after onset of disease. In patients with type 2 diabetes, screening should begin at the time of diagnosis.

1. Easiest in-office screening method

   Measure albumin-to-creatinine ratio in a random spot collection.

   First void or other morning collections are preferred because of the known diurnal variation in albumin excretion.

2. 24-hour creatinine collection
3. Timed collection (4 hours or overnight)

If assays for microalbuminuria are not readily available, screen with reagent tablets or dipsticks. However, despite their acceptable sensitivity (95%) and specificity (93%), all positive test findings should be confirmed by more specific methods.

PREVENTION AND TREATMENT[22]

Once microalbuminuria is detected, the clinical goals should be improvement in glucose control, adherence to low-protein diets, and treatment of co-existing hypertension if present. In many cases, microalbuminuria may be present yet the blood pressure may be considered normal or near normal. In such cases, the addition of an ACE inhibitor may markedly reduce the microalbuminuria.

To prevent nephropathy, help patients to do the following:

- Maintain tight glycemic control

- Strive for reduction in protein intake
- Control hypertension (ACE inhibitors have proven effective in preventing the progression of kidney disease; further research is required regarding the roles of other antihypertensive agents in this process)
- Lower cholesterol and lose weight

■ Neuropathy[23,24]

DIFFUSE PERIPHERAL NEUROPATHY

The most common type of peripheral neuropathy creates bilateral damage to the nerves of the extremities, especially the feet. At least 15% of all people with diabetes eventually develop a foot ulcer; 6 of every 1,000 such patients undergo amputation. (Once amputation of one limb has occurred, prognosis for the contralateral limb is poor.) However, nearly 75% of all amputations caused by neuropathy and poor circulation could be prevented with careful foot care (see section below).[23]

Symptoms

- Numbness or insensitivity to pain or temperature
- Tingling, burning, or prickling
- Sharp pains or cramps
- Extreme sensitivity to touch
- Loss of balance and coordination

Note: These symptoms are often worse at night.

If not recognized and aggressively treated, neuropathy may progress to the following:

- Loss of reflexes
- Muscle weakness
- A widened, shortened foot
- Gait changes and foot ulcers as patient places pressure on different parts of the feet

Note: Injuries may go unnoticed and become infected because of the patient's loss of sensation. If ulcers or foot injuries are not treated in time, infection may involve the bone and require amputation.

DIFFUSE AUTONOMIC NEUROPATHY

Diffuse neuropathy can hinder the body's normal response to hypoglycemia and affect a broad range of systems. This could result in a patient's inability to recognize and treat an insulin reaction. This disorder also interferes with proper functioning of the sweat glands and ability to regulate body temperature. Profuse night sweats and gustatory sweating can also occur.

Symptoms Related to Digestion

- Severe gastroparesis with persistent nausea, vomiting, bloating, loss of appetite, weight loss, large fluctuations of blood glucose
- Difficulty swallowing, if esophageal nerves are involved
- Constipation or frequent diarrhea, especially at night, with nerve damage to the bowels

Symptoms Related to Urinary Function and Male Sexual Response

See Bladder Dysfunction, page 135, and Impotence, page 136.

FOCAL NEUROPATHY

Focal neuropathy occurs most frequently in older patients with mild diabetes. Typically, specific nerves are affected, most often in the torso, leg, or head, and onset of symptoms is generally sudden. Pain tends to resolve on its own after a period of weeks or months, without causing long-term damage.[23]

Symptoms

- Pain in chest, stomach, flank, or front of the thigh
- Severe pain in the lower back or pelvis
- Pain in the chest or abdominal pain sometimes mistaken for angina, heart attack, or appendicitis
- Aching behind an eye
- Inability to focus the eye
- Double vision
- Bell's palsy
- Difficulty hearing

NEUROPATHY DIAGNOSIS

A careful evaluation of the legs and feet should be performed annually. The overall physical examination of the patient will test muscle strength, reflexes, sensitivity to position, vibration, temperature, and light touch. Nerve conduction studies should be performed to check the flow of electrical current through a nerve if the diagnosis is in question. Impulses that seem slower or weaker than usual indicate possible damage to the nerve. Electromyography, usually done in conjunction with nerve conduction studies, checks muscle response and electrical activity. Again, a slowed response suggests damage.

American Diabetes Association Clinical Practice Recommendations*

- Check between the toes and the posterior aspect of the heels (skin and nail deformities are a risk factor for development of foot ulcers or infection).
- Evaluate quantitative somatosensory threshold using the Semmes Weinstein monofilament or vibratory sensation.
- Palpate the pulses in the lower extremities and inspect for any gross ischemic changes.
- Check foot and ankle joint range of motion and inspect for bone abnormalities.
- Observe the patient for abnormal gait or stance (with and without shoes) and abnormal wear pattern of shoes.

In the presence of a cutaneous ulceration

- Measure the ulcer's size, depth, and structure
- Examine for purulent exudate, necrosis, sinus tracts, and odor
- Assess surrounding tissue for signs of edema, cellulitis, abscess, and fluctuation
- Exclude systemic infection
- Perform a vascular evaluation
- Conduct a radiologic examination, bone biopsy, or additional imaging studies if there is suspicion of advanced pathology

PREVENTION AND TREATMENT

Pain

Standard over-the-counter medications can be used to relieve pain. In patients with renal disease, nonsteroidal anti-inflammatory drugs should be used with caution. Topical cream containing cap-

---

*Adapted from American Diabetes Association,[24] with permission.

saicin may also be useful. In addition, the analgesic tramadol (Ultram) is an acceptable prescription pain medication.

Antidepressants such as amitriptyline (sometimes used with fluphenazine), carbamazepine, or phenytoin sodium have been used to reduce painful neuropathy; whereas some patients report a benefit, a significant clinical effect is not seen in many other patients. Codeine can be prescribed for short-term use to relieve severe pain.

Nonpharmacologic treatment for pain includes transcutaneous electrical nerve stimulation (TENS), hypnosis, relaxation training, biofeedback, and acupuncture. Walking regularly and wearing nonconstricting elastic stockings may help relieve leg pain. Warm (not hot) baths and massage may also relieve pain.

Gastrointestinal Problems

To ease mild symptoms of gastric stasis, advise patients to eat small, frequent meals and avoid fat. Less fiber may also help. For severe gastroparesis, metoclopramide can help speed digestion and relieve nausea. Erythromycin may also be beneficial for gastroparesis. To relieve diarrhea associated with bacterial overgrowth due to stasis, antibiotics such as tetracycline may be used.

Dizziness and Weakness

Patients should be advised to sit and stand slowly. When lying down, they should raise the head of the bed. Physical therapy can help to correct muscle weakness or loss of coordination. The use of nonconstricting elastic stockings can also be of help to the patient. Increasing salt in the diet in the absence of hypertension may relieve dizziness and weakness. (Salt-retaining hormones such as fludrocortisone can be used.)

Foot Ulcers[24]

Because bacterial infections of foot lesions are commonly polymicrobial, a suspected infection should be treated immediately with broad-spectrum antibiotics. Modify the treatment as necessary on the basis of culture results.

Culture by swab technique may be misleading. Rather, sterile saline irrigation of necrotic tissue, followed by curettage of the base of the ulceration, is recommended.

Incise and drain all abscessed infections. Debridement must extend to viable noninfected tissue. Although several topical agents such as antiseptic solutions have been proposed to speed healing, no adequately controlled studies have been conducted to evaluate their efficacy.

Good blood glucose control and proper nutritional status will aid in the healing process. Patients who heal slowly and inadequately may exhibit decreased pulses and/or pressures. This can be confirmed through Doppler examination. Such patients may be candidates for vascular reconstruction.

Minimize weight bearing on the ulcer. Bed rest, crutches, total-contact casts, shoe inserts, and special shoes are part of treatment. All patients on bed rest should have heel and ankle protection, and both legs should be inspected daily. Vasodilator drugs have not been shown to heal diabetic foot ulcers, and vasoconstrictor drugs should be avoided.

To prevent foot ulcers, advise patients to have feet examined by a podiatrist or physician at least twice a year. The patient should be encouraged to check feet daily and report nonhealing sores or breaks to the physician. Patients should be provided information on general foot care; such information is available from the podiatrist or from the American Diabetes Association. Also, make sure patients understand that their specific medical and behavioral regimen to lower blood glucose, blood pressure, and cholesterol, along with smoking cessation, may aid in improving or maintaining vascular flow to the lower extremities.

Bladder Dysfunction[25]

Diabetic neuropathy affects the genitourinary system, where clinical symptoms usually manifest in patients who have had diabetes for more than 10 years. The range of voiding dysfunctions is referred to as diabetic cystopathy. Typically, bladder capacity increases to > 1,000 ml, postvoid residual urine increases to > 200 ml, and bladder contractility decreases (voiding pressure < 40 cm H_2O).

Symptoms
- Poor urinary stream; the sensation that the bladder is still partly full
- Straining to void; dribbling, hesitancy, and recurring infections
- Infrequent voiding

Diagnosis
If a patient experiences more than two urinary tract infections per year or signs of bladder dysfunction, check for bladder outlet obstruction (prostatic hypertrophy), perform cystometrography, or do both.

Treatment
Patients should urinate approximately every 4 hours, whether they feel the urge or not. Diminished bladder contraction in parasympathetic efferent neuropathy can be treated with bethanechol, 10 to 30 mg, three times a day. In more severe cases, an internal sphincter resection may be necessary. Severe sympathetic efferent neuropathy may require catheterization.

Impotence[25,26]

Impotence affects at least half—perhaps up to 60%—of all men with diabetes. Diabetic men tend to develop impotence some 10 to 15 years earlier than the general population.

Symptoms
- Gradual onset of impotence, with progressive severity
- Fewer and less rigid erections; eventually patient may not be able to sustain erection
- Libido usually does not change

- Psychological problems (anxiety, depression) occur
- Psychologically induced dysfunction may occur as a result of fear of impotence

Diagnosis

Eliminate the possibility of psychological impotence, indicated by sudden onset and/or complaints specific to a certain incident. Measure nocturnal erections with commercially available devices. A man with intact neural and vascular mechanisms will have several erections during sleep. Doppler ultrasound can be used to measure penile blood supply. Venous leaks can be detected using penile sonography.

Treatment

Patients may avoid vascular and neuropathic complications by quitting smoking, decreasing alcohol, and maintaining tight glucose control. If the physician suspects that the patient's impotence is drug related, the patient's medication regimen may need to be altered. Injection of prostaglandins into the penis has been shown to be beneficial in a large percentage of men with diabetes. Newer therapies involve oral agents and penile suppositories. In particular, sildenafil (Viagra) has been shown to be very useful for treating erectile dysfunction in diabetic men. Testosterone injections may also help if hormone deficiency is the etiology. (This treatment, however, is not appropriate for older men at risk for prostate cancer.)

Vascular surgery can increase blood flow in the penis or repair venous leaks. Vacuum pumps can create an erection or a patient can have a penile implant.

If the impotence is psychological in origin, refer the patient to a qualified therapist.

Sexual Dysfunction in Women[25]

Older women with type 2 diabetes are more likely to experience sexual disorders (low desire, poor vaginal lubrication, dyspareunia, and difficulty reaching orgasm), possibly because of impaired genital vasocongestive response.

Diagnosis
Patients should be questioned regarding changes in sexual experience, such as

- Vaginal dryness or tightness with intercourse
- Pain or discomfort with intercourse, pain at penetration, with deep thrusting, or soreness after sexual activity
- Difficulty reaching orgasm
- Repeated vaginal or urinary infections

Treatment
Replacement estrogen in the form of pill, patch, or vaginal cream can improve vaginal elasticity and lubrication. Premenopausal women with diabetes can use nonprescription lubricants such as K-Y Jelly or Replens. To reduce coital pain, women can learn to relax the pubococcygeal muscles. Difficulty reaching orgasm may be related more to physical discomfort during sex than diabetic neuropathy.

Poor bladder control can interfere with sexual pleasure. Suggest to your patient that she empty her bladder before or within half an hour after intercourse. This will also help her avoid bladder infection. Concerns about pregnancy can interfere with sexual pleasure. Help your patient address these issues either with information on birth control (see Diabetes and Female Reproductive Health, page 140) or referral to a fertility specialist. In the case of intractable sexual problems, consider referring your patient to a mental health professional qualified to treat sexual problems.

Both men and women with diabetes may have to test their blood glucose and make necessary adjustments before engaging in sexual activity to avoid hypoglycemia afterward.

■ Skin Disorders and Infections

High glucose levels can put people with diabetes at greater risk of cutaneous disorders and a variety of infections. Drug therapy and tighter glycemic control can effectively manage some conditions. However, often there is no effective treatment; some disorders resolve spontaneously. The most commonly encountered skin disorders and infections are listed in Table 8-3.

TABLE 8-3 Most Commonly Encountered Skin Disorders and Infections[27]
Acanthosis nigricans
Scleroderma-like syndrome
Limited joint mobility
Scleroderma
Bacterial infections (e.g., malignant external otitis, necrotizing fasciitis)
Fungal and yeast infections (e.g., dermatophytosis, vaginal yeast infections)
Eruptive xanthomas
Necrobiosis lipoidica
Complications at injection sites
Gangrene
Oral diseases

■ Diabetes and Female Reproductive Health

MENSTRUATION

A week or so before the onset of the menstrual period, increased levels of estrogen and progesterone can affect blood glucose control. Advise patients to do the following[26]:

- Chart blood glucose levels to document fluctuations related to menstruation
- Chart PMS symptoms
- Eat and exercise regularly

If blood glucose before menstruation remains *higher* than normal, advise patients to do the following:

- Add extra exercise to the daily regimen
- Avoid eating extra carbohydrates
- Consider adding 1 to 2 additional units of insulin, returning to regular dose as soon as menstruation begins

If blood glucose before menstruation remains *lower* than normal, advise patients to do the following:

- Increase carbohydrate intake, adding healthy, low-fat foods
- Consider gradually decreasing insulin a few days before menstruation begins

For women with irregular periods and unpredictable glucose fluctuations, suggest they chart their ovulation to predict onset of menstruation by using basal body temperature records or an ovulation prediction kit, available over the counter.

MENOPAUSE[26]

Patients may experience greater insulin resistance during menopause because of hormonal changes and changes in body composition. Menopausal patients need to be even more vigilant about glycemic control and developing complications. When considering hormone replacement therapy, take into account risks and benefits that accrue to all menopausal women.

BIRTH CONTROL[26]

When choosing a birth control method, other than barrier techniques, consider the effect of hormones on blood glucose levels. Regardless of the chosen method, advise patients to do the following:

- Test blood glucose levels frequently, especially during the first few months; a small increase in insulin may be necessary

- Check glycated hemoglobin, blood pressure, cholesterol, and triglyceride levels 3 months after initiating oral contraceptives, and then at regular intervals thereafter

- Note that progesterone-containing intrauterine devices (IUDs) can increase a woman's risk of vaginal infections[28]

PRECONCEPTION PLANNING

Without good glycemic control at conception and during pregnancy, the fetus has a much-increased risk of developing birth defects; the mother runs a higher risk of hypertension and exacerbation of pre-existing diabetic complications. With careful monitoring and prenatal care, however, patients can avoid these problems. Ideally, patients should defer conception until an initial evaluation is completed and the therapy goals suggested below have been achieved. The ADA recommends the following preconception guidelines.*

Physical Examination

Potential risks for pregnancy-related complications require special emphasis on the following tests and procedures:

- Blood pressure measurement, including orthostatic changes
- Dilated retinal examination by an ophthalmologist or optometrist with experience managing diabetic retinopathy
- Cardiovascular examination, including electrocardiogram in patients with diabetes for more than 10 years or with other CHD risk factors
- Neurologic assessment, including autonomic function if necessary
- Examination of the lower extremities for evidence of vascular disease, neuropathy, deformity, or infection
- Pelvic examination, including Pap smear

Laboratory Evaluation

Critically important tests should be performed before conception to evaluate metabolic control and the presence of complications or related disease. These tests should include the following:

- Glycated hemoglobin
- Baseline assessment of renal function taken before conception and at regular intervals during pregnancy
- Thyroid function tests (including TSH)

Management Plan

An appropriate diet, including sufficient intake of folic acid and other vitamins and iron, should be instituted. Women with type

---

*Adapted from American Diabetes Association,[29] with permission.

2 diabetes should be switched to insulin therapy because the safety of oral agents during pregnancy has not been established. Self-monitoring of blood glucose should be kept at the following levels:

- Preprandial whole blood glucose: 70–100 mg/dl (3.9–5.6 mmol/L); or plasma glucose: 80–110 mg/dl (4.4–6.1 mmol/L)
- Postprandial whole blood glucose: 1 h < 140 mg/dl (< 7.8 mmol/L), 2 h < 120 mg/dl (< 6.7 mmol/L); or plasma glucose: 1 h < 155 mg/dl (< 8.6 mmol/L, 2 h < 135 mg/dl (< 7.5 mmol/L)

The goal for the glycated hemoglobin values should be within or near the upper limit of the normal laboratory reading or within 3 standard deviations of the normal mean. These goals may be modified depending on the patient's ability to recognize hypoglycemia and the risk of severe neuroglycopenia. Glycated hemoglobin tests should be repeated every 6 to 8 weeks until conception. (After 1 year, if your patient has not conceived, you may wish to refer her to a fertility specialist.)

Thoroughly evaluate, test, and stabilize hypertension, retinopathy, renal dysfunction, gastroparesis, and other neuropathies. Avoid using antihypertensive agents unsafe for pregnancy (ACE inhibitors, beta-blockers, and diuretics).

■ In-Hospital Care for Patients With Diabetes*

An estimated three million people are admitted to US hospitals every year for diabetes-related problems. The ADA suggests that inpatient care may be appropriate in the following situations[30]:

---

*Adapted from American Diabetes Association,[30] with permission.

- Life-threatening acute metabolic complications of diabetes:

  Diabetic ketoacidosis with blood glucose > 250 mg/dl (> 13.9 mmol/L) with arterial pH < 7.30 or serum bicarbonate level < 18 mEq/L; and ketonuria and/or ketonemia

  Hyperosmolar nonketotic state: impaired mental status and elevated plasma osmolality ($\geq$ 320 mOsm/kg; $\geq$ 320 mmol/kg) in patient with hyperglycemia ($\geq$ 600 mg/dl; $\geq$ 33.3 mmol/L)

  Hypoglycemia with neuroglycopenia when blood glucose < 50 mg/dl (< 2.8 mmol/L) and the treatment of hypoglycemia has not resulted in prompt recovery of sensorium; if the patient lapses into coma, or if seizures or altered behavior exists; if the patient will be alone for the next 12 hours even if the hypoglycemia has been treated; or if the hypoglycemia was caused by a sulfonylurea drug with a prolonged half-life

- Newly diagnosed diabetes in children and adolescents
- Substantial and chronic poor metabolic control that necessitates close monitoring of the patient to determine the cause of the problem and to modify therapy for at least one of the following:

  Hyperglycemia associated with volume depletion

  Persistent refractory hyperglycemia associated with metabolic deterioration

  Recurring fasting hyperglycemia > 300 mg/dl (> 16.7 mmol/L) that is refractory to outpatient therapy or a HbA$_{1c}$ level $\geq$ 100% above the upper limit of normal

  Recurring episodes of severe hypoglycemia (i.e., < 50 mg/dl [< 2.8 mmol/L]) despite intervention

  Metabolic instability manifested by frequent swings between hypoglycemia (< 50 mg/dl [< 2.8 mmol/L]) and fasting hyperglycemia (> 300 mg/dl [> 16.7 mmol/L])

Recurring diabetic ketoacidosis without precipitating infection or trauma

Repeated absence from school or work due to severe psychosocial problems that cannot be managed on an outpatient basis

- Severe chronic complications that require intensive treatment or severe conditions unrelated to diabetes that significantly affect its control or are affected by diabetes

- Uncontrolled or newly discovered insulin-requiring diabetes during pregnancy

- Institution of insulin-pump therapy or other intensive insulin regimens

SOME NOTES OF CAUTION

The sliding scale insulin regimen, used in an estimated 75% of all diabetic patients in US hospitals, has been reported to be ineffective in many cases and potentially dangerous.[31] Keeping patients on whatever standard insulin regimen has been effective at home and modifying that regimen according to patient response to treatment is advised.

When patients are admitted for reasons unrelated to diabetes, quality care requires a physician-led team with expertise in diabetes working with the physician responsible for the patient's intercurrent illness.

■ References

1. American Diabetes Association. Clinical Practice Recommendations 2000. Diabetic retinopathy. *Diabetes Care.* 2000;23(suppl 1):S73–S76.
2. American Diabetes Association. Clinical Practice Recommendations 2000. Management of dyslipidemia in adults with diabetes. *Diabetes Care.* 2000; 23(suppl 1):S57–S60.

3. Goldberg RB. Cardiovascular disease in diabetic patients. *Med Clin North Am.* 2000;84(1):81–93.

4. Howard BV, Robbins DC, Sievers ML, et al. LDL cholesterol as a strong predictor of coronary heart disease in diabetic individuals with insulin resistance and low LDL: The Strong Heart Study. *Arterioscler Thromb Vasc Biol.* 2000; 20:830–835.

5. Scandinavian Simvastatin Survival Study Group. Randomised trial of cholesterol lowering in 4444 patients with coronary heart disease: the Scandinavian Simvastatin Survival Study (4S). *Lancet.* 1994;344:1383–1389.

6. Sacks FM, Moye LA, Davis BR, et al. Relationship between plasma LDL concentrations during treatment with pravastatin and recurrent coronary events in the Cholesterol and Recurrent Events Trial. *Circulation* 1998;97:1446–1452.

7. Shepard J, Cobbe SM, Ford I, et al. Prevention of coronary heart disease with pravastatin in men with hypercholesterolemia. *N Engl J Med.* 1995;333: 1301–1307.

8. Downs JR, Clearfield M, Weis S, et al. Primary prevention of acute coronary events with lovastatin in men and women with average cholesterol levels: results of AFCAPS/TexCAPS. *JAMA.* 1998;279:1615–1622.

9. Pyorala K, Pedersen TR, Kjekshus J, et al. Cholesterol lowering with simvastatin improves prognosis of diabetic patients with coronary heart disease: a subgroup analysis of the Scandinavian Simvastatin Survival Study (4S). *Diabetes Care.* 1997;20:614.

10. Goldberg RB, Mellies MJ, Sacks FM, et al. Cardiovascular events and their reduction with pravastatin in diabetic and glucose-intolerant myocardial infarction survivors with average cholesterol levels: subgroup analyses in the Cholesterol and Recurrent Events (CARE) Trial. *Circulation.* 1998;98:13–19.

11. Benlian P, Cansier C, Hennache G, et al. Comparison of a new method for the direct and simultaneous assessment of LDL- and HDL-cholesterol with ultracentrifugation and established methods. *Clin Chem.* 2000;46:493–505.

12. American Diabetes Association. Consensus Statement: Detection and management of lipid disorders in diabetes. *Diabetes Care.* 1993;16:828–834.

13. Maron D, Fazio S, Linton MF. Current perspectives on statins. *Circulation.* 2000;101:207.

14. Arch J, Korytkowski M. Strategies for preventing coronary heart disease in diabetes mellitus. *Diabetes Spectrum.* 1999;12:88–94.

15. Hulley S, Grady D, Bush T, et al. Randomized trial of estrogen plus progestin for secondary prevention of coronary heart disease in postmenopausal women. *JAMA.* 1998;280:605–613.

16. Herrington DM, Reboussin DM, Brosnihan KB, et al. Effects of estrogen replacement on the progression of coronary-artery atherosclerosis. *N Engl J Med.* 2000;343:522–529.

17. American Diabetes Association. Clinical Practice Recommendations 2000. Standards of medical care for patients with diabetes mellitus. *Diabetes Care.* 2000;23(suppl 1):S32–S42.

18. United Kingdom Prospective Diabetes Study Group. Efficacy of atenolol and captopril in reducing risk of macrovascular and microvascular complications in type 2 diabetes: UKPDS 39. *BMJ.* 1998;317:713–720.

19. American Diabetes Association. Consensus Statement: Treatment of hypertension in diabetes. *Diabetes Care.* 1993;16:1394–1401.

20. Heart Outcomes Prevention Evaluation Study Investigators. Effects of ramipril on cardiovascular and microvascular outcomes in people with diabetes mellitus: results of the HOPE study and MICRO-HOPE substudy. *Lancet.* 2000;355: 253–259.

21. National Institute of Diabetes and Digestive and Kidney Diseases (NIDDK). Kidney Disease of Diabetes. Available at: http://www.niddk.nih.gov/health/kidney/pubs/kdd/kdd.htm#care. Accessed November 13, 2000.

22. American Diabetes Association. Clinical Practice Recommendations 2000. Diabetic nephropathy. *Diabetes Care.* 2000;23(suppl 1):S69–S72.

23. National Institute of Diabetes and Digestive and Kidney Diseases (NIDDK). Diabetic Neuropathy: The Nerve Damage of Diabetes. NIH Publication No. 95–3185, July 1995, updated October 1999. Available at http://www.niddk.nih.gov/health/diabetes/pubs/neuro/neuro.htm. Accessed August 11, 2000.

24. American Diabetes Association. Clinical Practice Recommendations 1998. Foot care in patients with diabetes mellitus. *Diabetes Care.* 1998;21(suppl 1).

25. Lebovitz HE, ed. *Therapy for Diabetes Mellitus and Related Disorders.* 2nd ed. Alexandria, Va: American Diabetes Association, 1994.

26. Kelley DB, ed-in-chief. *American Diabetes Association Complete Guide to Diabetes.* Alexandria, Va: American Diabetes Association; 1996.

27. Porte D Jr., Sherwin RS, eds. *Ellenberg & Rifkin's Diabetes Mellitus.* 5th ed. New York, NY: McGraw-Hill; 1997.

28. Hodoglugil NN, Aslan D, Bertan M. Intrauterine device use and some issues related to sexually transmitted disease screening and occurrence. *Conception.* 2000;61(6):359–364.

29. American Diabetes Association. Clinical Practice Recommendations 2000. Preconception care of women with diabetes. *Diabetes Care.* 2000;23(suppl 1):65–68.

30. American Diabetes Association. Clinical Practice Recommendations 2000. Hospital admission guidelines for diabetes mellitus. *Diabetes Care*. 2000. 23(suppl 1):S83.
31. Queale WS, Seidler AJ, Brancati FL. Glycemic control and sliding scale insulin use in medical inpatients with diabetes mellitus. *Arch Intern Med*. 1997;157: 545–552.

CHAPTER NINE

Leading-Edge Research

New Approaches to Prevention

Scientists continue to search for the causes of diabetes, for ways to prevent or cure the disease, and for better treatments. Even modest advances in the prevention of diabetes would have enormous impact. For example, if individuals with a 10% risk of developing type 2 diabetes each year reduced their risk to 8% per year, this risk reduction would prevent the occurrence of 7,000 to 9,000 person-years of blindness, renal failure, and amputation caused by diabetes.[1]

In the late 1990s, the NIDDK, in collaboration with other National Institutes of Health institutes and the private sector, funded two major primary-prevention trials, both of which are still in progress. More than 150,000 individuals will be screened when recruitment for these two studies is completed.[1]

The first trial, the Diabetes Prevention Trial—Type 1 (DPT-1), is a national, randomized, placebo-controlled study designed to investigate the possibility of preventing or delaying the onset of type 1 diabetes in individuals with immunologic markers for the disease. The study will investigate whether insulin can delay or prevent diabetes by altering the immune process that destroys β-cells. At more than 350 screening locations, relatives of patients with type 1 diabetes will be tested for antibodies involved in the immune destruction of β-cells. If antibodies and evidence of β-cell damage are detected, individuals will be randomly assigned to treatment with insulin injections. If antibodies and minimal β-cell damage is found, individuals will be randomized to oral insulin capsules.[1]

The second trial is the Diabetes Prevention Program (DPP), a national study designed to assess the possibility of preventing type 2 diabetes in high-risk individuals by means of drugs, diet, and exercise. In this study, risk is assessed based on blood glucose testing, age, family history, and medical history. High-risk individuals are targeted for study inclusion. Study participants undergo a glucose tolerance test to differentiate abnormal glucose tolerance from true diabetes. High-risk persons will be randomized to lifestyle changes with a placebo, more intensive lifestyle changes (weight loss and exercise), or an oral antidiabetic drug.

■ New Approaches to Restoring Insulin Secretion

PANCREATIC TRANSPLANTS

A physiologic approach to reversing diabetes is the transplantation of pancreatic insulin-secreting tissue. Transplantation presents a major opportunity for patients with end-stage renal disease to improve quality of life, obtain freedom from insulin injections, enhance glycemic control, and potentially increase survival. However, that opportunity comes with an increased risk of organ rejection, infection, and surgical complications, along with high financial cost and extended hospitalization. Lifelong immunosuppression to prevent rejection and a 2–3% risk of immunosuppression-related lymphoma are added considerations.[2]

An alternative to transplanting the entire pancreas is the transplantation of isolated islets of Langerhans. It has been demonstrated that islet cell transplants can provide glycemic control and reverse insulin dependence. Researchers at the University of Alberta recently reported on the successful transfer of human pancreatic islet cells into seven patients with type 1 diabetes. The transplantation was done by injection into the liver via the portal vein, eliminating the need for surgery. A steroid-free combination of the drugs tacrolimus, sirolimus, and daclizumab was used to prevent cell rejection and the return of autoimmune diabetes. No clinical evidence of graft rejection was seen, and glycemic control was attained, along with freedom from insulin therapy.[3] These results hold the promise of life without dependence on insulin injections for patients with diabetes.

GENETICALLY ENGINEERING β-CELLS

Further contributing to optimism is recent research into the development of an in vitro line of human β-cells. The cells have successfully produced insulin in vitro and in lab animals. This development may lead to an unconstrained source of β-cells for transplantation, overcoming the current shortage of cells obtained from organ donors.[4]

Metabolic control of insulin production is one of the major problems with genetic engineering of β-cells. However, researchers have found that pituitary cells have the same signaling pathways as the pancreatic β-cells for producing hormones and that pituitary cells survive in mice whose pancreatic β-cells are destroyed by the immune system. Through this research, scientists may clear the hurdle of regulating the release of insulin, if the peptide hormone GLP-1 turns out to have the same effect on pituitary cells as it does on β-cells. Secreted by the stomach, GLP-1 signals the pancreas when to release insulin. Another similar peptide may work as well.[5,6]

A gene for islet neogenesis-associated protein (*INGAP*) may convert dormant cells found on the pancreas into insulin-producing β-cells, another new approach considered for restoring insulin secretion. This could benefit patients with type 1 diabetes as well as those in the advanced stages of type 2 diabetes.[7]

GENE MAPPING AND GENE THERAPY

The Human Genome Project has as its goal the sequencing of all human genes. To understand the genesis of a disease, and therefore provide preventive strategies, all genes involved in the development of a disease and its complications must be identified. Genetic variations between individuals, known as polymorphisms, are used to identify disease-causing genes. Single nucleotide polymorphisms (SNPs) are useful genetic markers that occur frequently and can be measured with automated techniques. These techniques will provide vast amounts of information and valuable clues to the function of identified genes.[8] Long-term research in genetic engineering has the potential to aid in the development of fuel-responsive insulin-secreting human cell lines, methods of immunoprotection of transplanted cell lines, and gene therapy approaches for the treatment of diabetes and diabetes complications.[9] A number of genes involved in the growth and differentiation of β-cells have been identified.[10]

An international research team has identified genetic mutations that trigger early onset of type 2 diabetes, the so-called maturity-onset diabetes of the young (MODY). Mapping the genes responsible (*MODY1*, *MODY2*, and *MODY3* on chromosomes 20, 7, and 12, respectively,[11,12] and *NIDDM2*, which may be involved in adult-onset type 2 diabetes and may be a different allele of *MODY3*[13]) could lead to new treatment approaches.

Already, gene therapy in animals has opened an intriguing avenue for treatment of humans. At the University of Texas Southwestern Medical Center in Dallas, researchers injected a recombinant adenovirus with the leptin gene into healthy rats with normal body fat. The animals overproduced leptin, which caused them to selectively lose all fat but no lean body mass. While the rodents' insulin levels dropped by more than half, they did not develop diabetes.[14] The animals' sensitivity to insulin may be linked to body fat—the more fat, the less sensitive. These findings may offer some insight into the pathophysiology of insulin resistance in humans. In humans, higher leptin concentrations have been shown to be associated with higher body mass index, percentage body fat, and amount of abdominal adipose tissue as well as with a higher degree of insulin resistance.[15]

■ Advances in Insulin Therapy

Purdue University is developing a gel-like material that might someday be used to deliver insulin in a way that mimics the body's natural response to changing glucose levels in the blood. Expanding and contracting as the acidity in its environment changes, the gel could be used to make a "molecular gate" where high glucose levels would make the substance shrink away from both sides of a tiny pore. The pore would then open like a gate and allow molecules of insulin to pass through. The gel could be surgically inserted into the peritoneal cavity.[16]

So far, attempts at developing an oral formulation of insulin have failed because the insulin molecule is broken down in the gut. However, researchers at Brown University have met with some success in developing such a formulation. They encased insulin in small plastic beads fed to mice, where the insulin was successfully absorbed into the bloodstream.[17]

Implantable insulin pumps (IIPs) deliver insulin directly into the abdominal cavity and mimic natural insulin production better than subcutaneous injections. They have been shown to be associated with less variation in blood glucose levels and thus fewer episodes of hypoglycemia than multiple daily injections.[18,19] In addition, patients with IIP were more satisfied with their treatment and did not gain weight as they had on an intensive self-injection regimen.[18] Because of problems with insulin flow and clogging, the US Food and Drug Administration has not yet approved any IIP for use in the United States.

Another new approach intended to eliminate invasive injections is the insulin jet injector, which uses a high-pressure mechanism to send a fine spray of insulin directly through the skin, eliminating the need for needles.[20]

Other novel insulin delivery systems under consideration include the inhaled insulin devices. Several systems currently under development show great promise and may be available for use by patients with both type 1 and type 2 diabetes in just a few years. Results of preliminary studies with these new delivery systems have dismissed concerns about variability of drug administration,[21,22] and the efficacy and safety of these formulations appear to be equivalent to that of regular insulin. For example, pharmacokinetic studies have shown that a dry-powder formulation of insulin has the following effects: a faster onset of action than subcutaneous regular insulin, a duration of action between that for subcutaneous regular insulin and subcutaneous insulin lispro, and a time to peak effect similar to that for subcutaneous insulin lispro.[23] The safety and efficacy of this formulation were compared with conventional insulin in several 3-month studies. In two studies, one involving 70 patients with type 1 diabetes and another analyzing 51 patients with type 2 diabetes, patients were randomly assigned to conventional therapy (two to three injections per day) or an inhaled insulin group (premeal inhaled insulin and bedtime Ultralente injection). In type 1 patients, glycemic control, as measured via HbA_{1c}, did not differ, and 80% of the patients in the inhaled insulin group opted for a 1-year extension of therapy.[24] In the type 2 study, glycemic control, as measured by HbA_{1c}, did not differ, and satisfaction was high—92% of patients requested a 1-year extension of therapy with inhaled insulin.[25] Finally, in a study of 69 patients with type 2 diabetes in whom oral antihyperglycemic therapy had failed, continuation of oral therapy (sulfonylurea and/or metformin) was compared with a regimen of one oral agent plus inhaled insulin (one to two puffs three times before meals). Those patients receiving the inhaled insulin protocol showed a marked improvement in HbA_{1c} (–2%, $P < 0.0001$) compared with patients receiving oral therapy alone.[26] A 2-year extension study involving patients from the 3-month trials has shown that efficacy (based on HbA_{1c}) and pulmonary safety (as assessed with full pulmonary function tests and spirometry) in patients using inhaled insulin have been sustained during 24 months of therapy.[27]

Another novel insulin delivery system is a handheld device and dosage form that delivers standard liquid parenteral formulations of insulin, as fine aerosol droplets, deep into the lung.[28,29] In a recent randomized crossover study of 20 patients, the pharmacokinetic effects and safety of insulin given via this method were compared with those for subcutaneous regular insulin. Reproducible pharmacodynamic effects on blood glucose, similar to those with subcutaneous insulin, were seen with this inhaled product. Safety results were also comparable to those for standard insulin therapy.[22] In a randomized, open-label, five-period, crossover trial, the pharmacokinetic and pharmacodynamic profiles of this inhaled insulin were compared with those for subcutaneous insulin in C-peptide–negative type 1 diabetes patients. A dose-response relationship was seen for all pharmacokinetic and pharmacodynamic parameters measured after administration of inhaled insulin.[30]

Other formulations for inhaled insulin are also currently in development. In addition, a buccal formulation of insulin administered into the oral cavity as a fine spray is in clinical trials in North America and Europe.[31]

■ Research on Compounds

Identification of the obese gene (*OB*) and its product, leptin, have led to speculation regarding the potential effects of leptin on reversal of obesity, curbing of food intake, and acceleration of energy expenditure. Recent studies have shed light on the role leptin may play in the pathophysiology of obesity and diabetes. In a study investigating the effect of acute insulin deprivation and hyperinsulinemia on the plasma leptin levels of patients with type 1 diabetes and healthy individuals, acute insulin deprivation reduced plasma leptin in patients with type 1 diabetes. However, hyperinsulinemia was found to significantly reduce leptin levels in healthy women and had no effect on plasma leptin levels in healthy men. The effects of acute hyperinsulinemia on plasma leptin were found to be gender dependent, and basal insulin was found to have a role in regulating postabsorptive leptin levels.[32] In a study involving 45 patients with type 2 diabetes and 60 healthy individuals, gender and fat mass were found to be independent predictors of leptin, with gender accounting for 33% of the total leptin variance.[33]

■ Glucose-Monitoring Technology

For 30 years, scientists have tried to perfect an implantable glucose sensor. Several types of devices remain under study, including hydrogen peroxide–based enzyme electrode sensors, oxygen-based sensors, and membrane-covered catalytic electrodes.[34]

Given the importance of glucose monitoring, development of a noninvasive blood glucose monitoring system has obvious import, because it would spare patients from having to prick their fingers multiple times a day to maintain tight control. The types of devices and methods in development include shining infrared light through a forearm or finger, drawing glucose from the blood up through the skin using a low-level electric current, and measuring glucose in saliva or tears.[35]

One of these monitoring systems records tissue glucose levels using a glucose sensor. The sensing mechanism is inserted, like a tiny needle, under the skin of the abdomen. The sensor reads glucose levels in the interstitial fluid at 5-minute intervals for up to 3 days. During the monitoring process, the patient needs to calibrate the meter using a standard fingerstick measurement and five additional meter fingerstick measurements each day, to calculate glucose sensor values. The system monitor, connected to the sensor, collects up to 72 hours' worth of data that is then downloaded by the physician's office. The information can then be reviewed by the patient together with the physician and used in the development of a disease management strategy.[36,37]

Another very promising minimally invasive blood glucose monitoring device looks similar to a wristwatch and is worn on the forearm. It checks blood sugar levels every 20 minutes by sending tiny electric currents though the skin to extract interstitial fluid. The glucose level in the fluid is measured electrochemically. An alarm sounds when blood glucose levels become dangerously high or low. Studies have shown that this device gives accurate blood glucose readings when compared to the current fingerstick method of testing.[38]

In the recent past, technology has also succeeded in providing the patient with the ability to monitor objective glycemic control with blood tests that were at one time available only in clinical laboratories. Specifically, home glucose meters that record fructosamine levels (a measure of serum glycated proteins that objectively reflects antecedent glycemia for the preceding 1 to 3 weeks)[39] have recently been made available. As stated in Chapter 4, this home test may greatly aid the patient in efforts to normalize glycemic levels.

■ References

1. Diabetes Research Working Group. Diabetes research programs funded by the NIH. In: *Conquering Diabetes: A Strategic Plan for the 21st Century*. Bethesda, Md: National Institutes of Health, National Institute of Diabetes and Digestive and Kidney Diseases; 1999:47–53. Available at: http://www.niddk.nih.gov/federal/dwg/fr.pdf. Accessed September 21, 2000.

2. Ryan EA. Pancreas transplants: for whom? [commentary]. *Lancet*. 1998;351:1072–1073.

3. Shapiro AMJ, Lakey JRT, Ryan EA, et al. Islet transplantation in seven patients with type 1 diabetes mellitus using a glucocorticoid-free immunosuppressive regimen. *N Engl J Med*. 2000;343:230–238.

4. American Diabetes Association. Breakthrough research unveiled at ADA's 60th annual scientific sessions. Available at: http://www.diabetes.org/volunteervoice/summer2000/breakthrough.asp. Accessed August 18, 2000.

5. Lipes MA, Cooper EM, Skelly R, et al. Insulin-secreting non-islet cells are resistant to autoimmune destruction. *Proc Natl Acad Sci*. 1996;93:8595–8600.

6. Lipes MA, Davalli AM, Cooper EM. Genetic engineering of insulin expression in nonislet cells: implications for β-cell replacement therapy for insulin-dependent diabetes mellitus [review]. *Acta Diabetol*. 1997;34:2–5.

7. Gagliardino JJ, Del Zotto H, Massa L, et al. Sucrose administration to normal hamsters induces simultaneous changes in islet neogenesis and INGAP-positive cell mass. Presented at: American Diabetes Association 59th Annual Meeting and Scientific Sessions; June 19–22, 1999; San Diego, Calif. Abstract #1956.

8. Diabetes Research Working Group. Extraordinary research opportunities. In: *Conquering Diabetes: A Strategic Plan for the 21st Century*. Bethesda, Md: National Institutes of Health, National Institute of Diabetes and Digestive and Kidney Diseases; 1999:56–79. Available at: http://www.niddk.nih.gov/federal/dwg/fr.pdf. Accessed September 21, 2000.

9. Diabetes Research Working Group. Special needs for special problems. In: *Conquering Diabetes: A Strategic Plan for the 21st Century*. Bethesda, Md: National Institutes of Health, National Institute of Diabetes and Digestive and Kidney Diseases; 1999:80–96. Available at: http://www.niddk.nih.gov/federal/dwg/fr.pdf. Accessed September 21, 2000.

10. Leibowitz G, Levine F. Gene therapy for type 1 and type 2 diabetes. *Diabetes Rev*. 1999;7:124–138.

11. Yamagata K, Oda N, Kaisaiki PJ, et al. Mutations in the hepatocyte nuclear factor-1 alpha gene in maturity-onset diabetes of the young. *Nature*. 1996;384:455–458.

12. Yamagata K, Furuta H, Oda N, et al. Mutations in the hepatocyte nuclear factor-4 alpha gene in maturity-onset diabetes of the young. *Nature.* 1996;384:458–460.

13. Mahtani MM, Widen E, Lehto M, et al. Mapping of a gene for type 2 diabetes associated with an insulin secretion defect by a genome scan in Finnish families. *Nat Genet.* 1996;14:90–94.

14. Chen G, Koyama K, Yuan X, et al. Disappearance of body fat in normal rats induced by adenovirus-mediated leptin gene therapy. *Proc Natl Acad Sci.* 1996; 93:14795–14799.

15. Johannsson G, Karlsson C, Lonn L, et al. Serum leptin concentration and insulin sensitivity in men with abdominal obesity. *Obes Res.* 1998;6:416–421.

16. Dorski CM, Doyle FJ, Peppas NA. Preparation of glucose-sensitive P (MAA-g-EG) hydrogels. *Polym Mater Sci Eng Proceed.* 1997;76:281–282.

17. Mathiowitz E, Jacob JS, Jong YS, et al. Biologically erodible microspheres as potential oral drug delivery systems. *Nature.* 1997;386:410–414.

18. Saudek CD, Duckworth WC, Giobbie-Hurder A, et al. Implantable insulin pump vs multiple-dose insulin for non-insulin-dependent diabetes mellitus: a randomized clinical trial. *JAMA.* 1996;276:1322–1327.

19. Dunn FL, Nathan DM, Scavini M, et al. Long-term therapy of IDDM with an implantable insulin pump. *Diabetes Care.* 1997;20:59–63.

20. National Diabetes Information Clearinghouse Web site. National Institutes of Health, National Institute of Diabetes and Digestive and Kidney Diseases. Devices for taking insulin. Available at: http://www.niddk.nih.gov/health/diabetes/summary/altins/altins.htm. Accessed August 14, 2000.

21. Patton JS, Bukar J, Nagrajan S. Inhaled insulin. *Adv Drug Delivery Rev.* 1999; 35:235–247.

22. Farr SJ, Kipnes M, Otulana B, et al. A comparison of the pharmacodynamic effects of inhaled insulin versus subcutaneous insulin in type 1 diabetic patients. Presented at: American Diabetes Association 59th Annual Meeting and Scientific Sessions; June 19–22, 1999; San Diego, Calif. Abstract #0410.

23. Heise T, Rave K, Bott S, et al. Time-action profile of an inhaled insulin preparation in comparison to insulin Lispro and regular insulin. Presented at: American Diabetes Association 60th Annual Meeting and Scientific Sessions; June 9–13, 2000; San Antonio, Tex. Abstract #39.

24. Skyler JS, Gelfand RA, Kourides IA. Treatment of type 1 diabetes mellitus with inhaled insulin: a 3-month, multicenter trial. Presented at: American Diabetes Association 58th Annual Meeting and Scientific Sessions; June 11–16, 1998; Chicago, Ill. Abstract #0236.

25. Cefalu WT, Gelfand RA, Kourides I. Treatment of type 2 diabetes mellitus with inhaled human insulin: a 3-month, multicenter trial. Presented at: American

Diabetes Association 58th Annual Meeting and Scientific Sessions; June 11–16, 1998; Chicago, Ill. Abstract #0237.

26. Weiss SR, Berger S, Cheng S, et al. Adjunctive therapy with inhaled human insulin in type 2 diabetic patients failing oral agents: a multicenter phase II trial. Presented at: American Diabetes Association 59th Annual Meeting and Scientific Sessions; June 19–22, 1999; San Diego, Calif. Abstract #0048.

27. Cefalu WT, Balagtas CC, Landschulz WH, Gelfand RA. Sustained efficacy and pulmonary safety of inhaled insulin during 2 years of outpatient therapy. Presented at: American Diabetes Association 60th Annual Meeting and Scientific Sessions; June 9–13, 2000; San Antonio, Tex. Abstract #0406.

28. Aradigm. Liquid formulation technology. Available at: http://www.aradigm.com/tech/liquid_form.html. Accessed September 18, 2000.

29. Doctor's Guide. Inhaled insulin may allow diabetics to control meal-time glucose levels. Available at: http://www.pslgroup.com/dg/24a96.htm. Accessed October 3, 2000.

30. Brunner GA, Balent B, Sendhofer G, et al. Pharmacokinetics and pharmacodynamics of inhaled versus subcutaneous insulin in subjects with type 1 diabetes—a glucose clamp study. Presented at: American Diabetes Association 60th Annual Meeting and Scientific Sessions; June 9–13, 2000; San Antonio, Tex. Abstract #308.

31. Generex Biotechnology Corp. Lilly and Generex sign agreement to develop buccal form of insulin [press release]. September 6, 2000. Available at: http://www.generex.com/section2/news.html. Accessed September 18, 2000.

32. Nair KS, Barazzoni R, Meek S, Abu-Lebdeh H, Moller N. Effects on plasma leptin of acute insulin deprivation in type 1 diabetic patients and physiologic hyperinsulinemia in non-diabetic men and women. Presented at: American Diabetes Association 59th Annual Meeting and Scientific Sessions; June 19–22, 1999; San Diego, Calif. Abstract #1334.

33. Carantoni M, Solini A, Passaro A, et al. Different predictors of plasma leptin levels in normoglycemic subjects and patients with type 2 diabetes. Presented at: American Diabetes Association 59th Annual Meeting and Scientific Sessions; June 19–22, 1999; San Diego, Calif. Abstract #1882.

34. Gough DA, Armour JC. Perspectives in diabetics: development of the implantable glucose sensor: what are the prospects and why is it taking so long? *Diabetes.* 1995;44:1005–1009.

35. National Institute of Diabetes and Digestive and Kidney Diseases. Noninvasive blood glucose monitors. Available at: http://www.niddk.nih.gov/health/diabetes/summary/noninmet/noninmet.htm. Accessed October 3, 2000.

36. Food and Drug Administration. FDA approves new glucose monitoring system for diabetics [press release]. June 16, 1999. Available at: http://www.fda.gov/bbs/topics/NEWS/NEW00682.html. Accessed October 3, 2000.

37. MiniMed. Frequently asked questions. Available at: http://www.minimed.com/files/cgms/spec_pg2.htm. Accessed September 19, 2000.
38. American Diabetes Association. Watch-like device will check body's sugar levels painlessly [press release]. June 22, 1999. Available at: http://www.diabetes.org/am99/pressreleases/watch.asp. Accessed October 10, 2000.
39. Cefalu WT, Wang ZQ, Redmon E, et al., Clinical validity of a self-test fructosamine in outpatient diabetic management. *Diabetes Technol Ther.* 1999;1:435–441.

Patient Resources

American Association of Diabetes Educators
100 West Monroe Street
Suite 400
Chicago, IL 60603-1901
Tel: (800) 338-3633 or (312) 424-2426
Fax: (312) 424-2427
Diabetes Educator Access Line: (800) TEAMUP4 (800-832-6874)
Home page: http://www.aadenet.org
A professional organization that can help individuals locate a diabetes educator in their community.

American Diabetes Association
The National Office
1701 North Beauregard Street
Alexandria, VA 22311
Tel: (800) DIABETES (800-342-2383) reaches an affiliate office in the state in which the call is placed
or (703) 549-1500 (National Office)
Home page: http://www.diabetes.org
The American Diabetes Association publishes many books and resources for health professionals and people with diabetes, including *Diabetes Forecast*, a monthly magazine for patients, and the journals *Diabetes*, *Diabetes Care*, and *Diabetes Spectrum*.

American Dietetic Association
216 W. Jackson Boulevard
Chicago, IL 60606-6995
Tel: (800) 877-1600 or (312) 899-0040
Home page: http://www.eatright.org
A professional organization that can help individuals locate a registered dietitian in their community.

American Heart Association
7272 Greenville Avenue
Dallas, TX 75231
Tel: (800) 242-8721
Home page: http://www.americanheart.org
A private, voluntary organization that distributes literature on heart disease and its prevention. Local affiliates can be found in the telephone directory.

American Amputation Foundation
P.O. Box 250218
Little Rock, AR 72225
Tel: (501) 666-2523
Peer counseling for new amputees. Has local chapters and lists support groups.

American Podiatric Medical Association (APMA)
9312 Old Georgetown Road
Bethesda, MD 20814-1698
Tel: (301) 571-9200
Fax: (301) 530-2752
E-mail: askapma@apma.org
Home page: http://www.apma.org
APMA Foot Care Information Center
Tel: (800) FOOT-CARE (800-366-8227)
APMA publishes materials for professionals and the public, includ-

ing a diabetes-specific booklet, *Your Podiatric Physician Talks About Diabetes.*

Impotence World Association/Impotence Institute of America
119 South Ruth Street
Maryville, TN 37803
Tel: (800) 669-1603 or (865) 379-2154
Home page: http://www.impotenceworld.org
Provides information and physician referral in each state.

Indian Health Service
National Diabetes Program
5300 Homestead Road NE
Albuquerque, NM 87110
Tel: (505) 248-4182
Fax: (505) 248-4188
Home page: http: www.ihs.gov
Provides information tailored to Native American and Alaska Native communities: general diabetes information, nutrition education materials, and professional resources.

Juvenile Diabetes Foundation International
120 Wall Street
New York, NY 10005
Tel: (800) JDF-CURE (800-533-2873) or (212) 785-9500
Fax: (212) 785-9595
E-mail: info@jdf.org
Home page: http://www.jdfcure.org
A private, voluntary organization that funds research on diabetes and promotes public awareness. Local chapters located across the country sponsor programs and fundraising activities. Information about local groups is available in telephone directories or from the national office.

National Diabetes Information Clearinghouse
1 Information Way
Bethesda, MD 20892-3560
Tel: (800) 860-8747 or (301) 654-3327
Fax: (301) 907-8906
E-mail: ndic@info.niddk.nih.gov
Home page: http://www.niddk.nih.gov/health/diabetes/ndic.htm
A program of the National Institute of Diabetes and Digestive and Kidney Diseases (NIDDK), the Federal Government's leading agency for diabetes research. The clearinghouse distributes a variety of publications to the public and to health care professionals.

National Eye Institute (NEI)
National Eye Health Education Program
2020 Vision Place
Bethesda, MD 20892-3655
Tel: (800) 869-2020 or (301) 496-5248
Fax: (301) 402-1065
E-mail: 2020@nei.nih.gov
Home page: http://www.nei.nih.gov
Provides materials related to diabetic eye disease and its treatment, including literature for patients, guides for health care professionals, and education kits for community health care workers and pharmacists.

National Kidney and Urologic Diseases Information Clearinghouse
3 Information Way
Bethesda, MD 20892-3580
Tel: (800) 891-5390 or (301) 654-4415
Fax: (301) 907-8906
E-mail: nkudic@info.niddk.nih.gov
Home page: http://www.niddk.nih.gov

A service of the NIDDK. Provides information about kidney and urologic diseases to the public, patients and their families, and health care professionals.

Office of Minority Health Resource Center
P.O. Box 37337
Washington, DC 20013-7337
Tel: (800) 444-6472
Fax: (301) 230-7198
Home page: http://www.omhrc.gov
Offers information, publications, referrals, etc., to African American, Asian, Hispanic/Latino, Native American/Alaska Native, and Pacific Islander populations.

Weight Control Information Network (WIN)
1 WIN Way
Bethesda, MD 20892-3665
Tel: (877) 946-4627 or (202) 828-1025
Fax: (202) 828-1028
E-mail: win@info.niddk.nih.gov
Home page: http://www.niddk.nih.gov
A service of the NIDDK. Provides fact sheets, pamphlets, reprints, consensus statements, reports, and literature searches on weight control, obesity, and weight-related nutritional disorders.

SPECIAL SERVICES

International Diabetic Athletes Association
1647 West Bethany Home Road #B
Phoenix, AZ 85015
Tel: (800) 898-IDAA (800-898-4322) or (602) 433-2113
Fax: (602) 433-9331
E-mail: idaa@diabetes-exercise.org

Home page: http://www.getnet.com/~idaa/
Provides pamphlets on diabetes and exercise.

Medic Alert Foundation
2323 Colorado Avenue
Turlock, CA 95382
Tel: (800) 432-5378 or (209) 669-2406
Fax: (209) 669-2495
Home page: http://www.medicalert.org
Supplies medical ID bracelets and maintains a 24-hour emergency
response center to respond to calls regarding members.

Pedorthic Footwear Association
7150 Columbia Gateway Drive Suite G
Columbia, MD 21046-1151
Tel: (800) 673-8447
Fax: (410) 381-1167
Home page: http://www.pedorthics.org
Provides information on Medicare coverage of therapeutic shoes
for people with diabetes.

**International Association for Medical
Assistance to Travelers**
417 Center Street
Lewiston, NY 14092
Tel: (716) 754-4883
Fax: (519) 836-3412
Home page: http://www.sentex.net/~iamat
Can provide a list of doctors in foreign countries who can speak
English and were either trained in North America or Great
Britain.

DIABETES SUPPLIES BY MAIL ORDER

American Medical Supplies and Equipment Inc.
Tel: (305) 592-3422
Fax: (305) 477-3250
Home page: http://www.amerimed.com

Diabetic Express
Tel: (800) 338-4656
Fax: (800) 474-8262
Home page: http://www.diabeticexpress.com

HealthLogs
Tel: (800) 220-7111
Home page: http://www.healthlogs.com

National Diabetic Pharmacies
Tel: (800) INSULIN (800-467-8546) or (540) 777-0000
(English and Spanish)
Home page: http://www.rev.net/~ndp/